The Management of Alzheimer's Disease

The Management of Alzheimer's Disease

Edited by

GORDON K. WILCOCK

Professor of Care of the Elderly, University of Bristol, UK

WRIGHTSON BIOMEDICAL PUBLISHING LTD
Petersfield, UK and Bristol, PA, USA

The front cover shows axial (left) and coronal (right) SPECT scans demonstrating reduced blood flow (arrows) in the temporal lobes of a patient suffering from Alzheimer's disease.

Copyright © 1993 by Wrightson Biomedical Publishing Ltd

Editorial Office:

Wrightson Biomedical Publishing Ltd
Ash Barn House, Winchester Road, Stroud,
Petersfield, Hampshire GU32 3PN, UK
Telephone: 0730 265647
Fax: 0730 260368

British Library Cataloguing in Publication Data
A catalogue record for this book is available from the British Library.

Library of Congress Cataloging in Publication Data
The management of Alzheimer's disease/edited by Gordon K. Wilcock.
   p. cm.
  Includes bibliographical references and index.
  ISBN 1-871816-20-3 (hbk)
  1. Alzheimer's disease, I. Wilcock, G.K. (Gordon K.)
  [DNLM: 1. Alzheimer's Disease–therapy. WM 220 M266 1898]
RC523.M35 1993
618.97'683106–dc20
DNLM/DLC
for Library of Congress   93-3404
                           CIP

ISBN 1 871816 20 3 ✓

Composition by Scribe Design, Gillingham, Kent
Printed in Great Britain by Biddles Ltd, Guildford.

Contents

Preface

The management of people with dementia is becoming an increasingly important problem as the numbers of the very old increase. Until recently most of the approaches to this challenge were general responses posed by the dilemma of looking after people with cognitive impairment, particularly elderly subjects, rather than being specifically aimed at the individual illnesses that cause dementia. We are now beginning to move away from this and investigate specific approaches in relation to specific illnesses, such as Alzheimer's disease. Much of this advance is the result of our greater understanding of the natural history of Alzheimer's disease and its neurochemical basis, and we are at the threshold of being able to treat pharmacologically some of the disease's manifestations.

It is likely that in the years to come therapy for Alzheimer's disease will extend beyond treatments that are based on the cholinergic hypothesis. For the time being however most attempts at management will have to be focused largely on treatments that are predominantly cholinergic in their conception, against the background of more general measures designed to cope with certain practical aspects of caring for a person with dementia.

The existence of some light at the end of the therapeutic tunnel indicates that this is an opportune time to bring together in one volume many of the different strands that are part of the caring process, both practical and pharmacological, in the context of an appreciation of the size of the problem and its practical implications to the community at large.

This volume is divided into five sections. The first covers the scale of the problem, contrasting the epidemiology of Alzheimer's disease with its implications for government. Practical aspects of diagnosis follow in the second section. An international dimension is added in the chapters that deal with management issues, and this section also covers the role of different professionals as well as exploring the difficult issue of depression in relation to Alzheimer's disease.

The social impact of Alzheimer's disease is viewed across a broad spectrum with contributions from Government-funded research, the private nursing home sector and the Alzheimer's Disease Society, bringing together viewpoints from the National Institute of Social Work, the private and the voluntary sector.

Finally, there is a glimpse into the future with an examination of the potential for the development of new therapeutic strategies, and an examination of the role of the pharmaceutical industry in this context.

This is intended to be a book that contains useful information for readers with a variety of interests, to each of whom the authors hope some of the chapters will be of immediate value, leaving others to be dipped into in the future as and when necessary.

GORDON K. WILCOCK

I

The Scale of the Problem

The Management of Alzheimer's Disease
Edited by Gordon K. Wilcock
©1993 Wrightson Biomedical Publishing Ltd

1

The Epidemiology of Alzheimer's Disease

JOHN R.M. COPELAND

Professor and Head of Liverpool University Department of Psychiatry and Director of The Institute of Human Ageing, Liverpool, UK

INTRODUCTION

For the first time in the long history of man it has become necessary to consider how society will cope with the increasing proportions of persons surviving to advanced age. Recent population statistics for industrialized countries show that the proportion of the very old, aged 85 and over, has steadily increased and will go on increasing well into the next century, most obviously for women. This happy event is due largely to the success of modern medicine in preventing neonatal deaths and in adding a mean five years of life to those who survive to over 70 years of age. At present, man seems to have an upper age limit not far beyond 110 years and up until now few individuals with a well documented date of birth have survived longer than this time, however well they have otherwise seemed. Whether such a lifespan is genetically programmed and difficult to change, or whether it is environmentally determined and open to modification is unknown. How this would be done with an environmental cause presumably so widespread is also difficult to determine. Whether attempts should be made to increase lifespan is a matter for ethical debate. Certainly, serious social problems might be foreseen if the lifespan were lengthened by a sizeable percentage. However, the aim of trying to preserve people in good health, physically and intellectually, until shortly before death is a laudable goal for Health and Social Services. In order to accomplish this, the many debilitating diseases which affect older age, many until recently confused with ageing itself, must be studied with a view to prevention, cure or in some degree ameliorating their long-term effects.

One of the most important of these debilitating conditions is dementia. Dementia is particularly important because although its prevalence is low until the age of 75, after that age it rises steeply. Prevalence is the measure of the proportion of people with a disease in a community at any one time. Incidence is the rate of new cases of the disease occurring over a given time, usually one year. Knowing the levels of morbidity present in a community is of importance to the purchasers of services who will also want to know the levels of behavioural disturbance and therefore the type and quantity of services required. For the scientist, prevalence is not such an interesting figure as incidence, as it is influenced by a number of factors which make comparisons between geographical localities difficult, such as migration in and out of an area, the rate of institutionalization and the effectiveness of medical interventions which alter mortality or speed of recovery. Thus, although it is exciting for the epidemiologist to find differences of prevalence between geographical areas it is because they suggest studies of incidence, which is not so easily affected by such matters. If there were true differences in incidence then these would lead to a search for risk factors and causal explanations. Sadly, it must be admitted that differences of this kind have been found for many diseases but the causes have still eluded discovery. Prevalence studies are comparatively cheap because they involve surveying a population only once. For incidence studies a population must be screened in the first stage, in order to eliminate existing cases, and reinterviewed in a second stage to identify those non-cases which have now become cases. A two-stage design is clearly twice as expensive as prevalence studies and therefore fewer incidence studies have been undertaken.

DEFINING ALZHEIMER'S DISEASE

One problem which has bedevilled epidemiology is how to define a case of illness in the community. Normally, doctors and other care professionals have their 'cases' chosen for them by the patients themselves and their relatives. The epidemiologist will discover them at an earlier stage. Not all illnesses in their milder forms can be clearly distinguished from normal behaviour. It is important therefore to develop a definition of a case which is useful for the purpose of the study as well as a reliable method for identifying it. Epidemiology, especially of the mental disorders, has been confused by the use of different case definitions and different methods of screening and identification, leading to uncertainty about whether discrepancies found between geographical areas are really due to differences in the proportions of illness present or to the definitions and methods used. This has proved a serious problem for studies of dementia in the community. It is even more difficult when attempts are made to divide dementia into its different types.

Sometimes we do not know sufficient about a condition to be able to set up clear definitions. The criteria for Alzheimer's disease, for example, in spite of recent attempts to define them, generally remain those of dementia as a whole after the known causes have been removed. Thus Alzheimer's disease is probably a rag bag of diagnoses. Even the pathology of Alzheimer's disease appears to lie on a continuum with that of normal brain, especially normal ageing brain. There is accumulating evidence to suggest that this rag bag does contain a number of conditions with similar pathology. Some investigators have pointed to Alzheimer's disease occurring earlier in life and characterized by speech and motor problems with a rapid course, and a later onset disease characterized mainly by gradual memory disturbance (Bondareff, 1983). To these diagnoses has recently been added Lewy body disease (McKeith *et al.*, 1992). Some centres have made informal claims for this to be the second most common cause of dementia after Alzheimer's disease.

PREVALENCE AND INCIDENCE OF ALZHEIMER'S DISEASE

There have been considerable efforts internationally to define dementia and in particular Alzheimer's disease for the purposes of research, and there is a strong movement to adopt standardized methods of assessment. It is therefore becoming increasingly possible to derive an agreed figure for the prevalence of dementia from modern studies. The classical survey was undertaken by Kay *et al.* (1964) in Newcastle, UK yielding a figure around 5% for moderate to severe dementia, with a further 5% for mild dementia. Recently, Kay (1991), reviewing some 19 studies of dementia, pointed out that there are still considerable differences in the levels of illness recorded even though methods and diagnostic criteria have improved. For example, he cited the study by Clarke *et al.* (1986) on subjects aged 75 and over in an English town, where a figure of 2.5% was recorded for dementia, while a study in Shanghai by Zhang *et al.* (1990) found a level of 12.3%. When comparing all subjects, including those living at home in the community and in institutions, Clarke *et al.* found a level of 4.5%, while in a similar study in Canada by Robertson *et al.* (1989) a figure of 15.9% is quoted. Are these real differences in the population or are they still differences due to method?

Recent studies in the United Kingdom have shown more consistent findings, for example Morgan *et al.* (1987) in Nottingham found 4.3% for dementia, and Livingstone *et al.* (1990) in London, 5.1%. O'Connor *et al.* (1989) in Cambridge, UK recorded 10.5% in subjects aged 75 and over, a figure not dissimilar to other studies for this age group. In those studies which have specifically considered Alzheimer's disease, levels are more varied. Hasegawa *et al.* (1986) in Japan recorded 1.6% for women and 0.6%

for men, against O'Connor *et al.* who found 7.3% for males living in Cambridge, UK and Sulkava *et al.* (1985) who found 9.2% for women in their study in Finland. There has, however, been some consistency, with figures between 3% and 5% for European studies of Alzheimer's disease. Most prevalence studies have shown a trend for women to preponderate over men although this has reached significant levels only in two studies (Kokmen *et al.*, 1989; Molsa *et al.*, 1982) in addition to the studies reported below. Jagger *et al.* (1992) re-examined dementia in the same geographical area as the Clarke *et al.* study using a standardized method, the Cambridge Mental Disorders of the Elderly schedule (CAMDEX) (Roth *et al.*, 1986). They reassessed moderate to severe dementia to be 3.4% in the 1981 study and 5.2% in the 1988 study.

The EURODEM group is an EC supported consortium comprising some of the studies mentioned above which has undertaken meta-analysis of existing studies as well as encouraging the use of a standard minimum data set. Examining the frequency and distribution of Alzheimer's disease diagnosed according to the *Diagnostic and Statistical Manual of the Mental Disorders (third edition, revised)* of the American Psychiatric Association (1990) and more specifically by the criteria of the National Institute of Neurological and Communicative Disorders and Stroke–Alzheimer's Disease and Related Disorders Association (McKhann *et al.*, 1984), they surveyed 23 European studies of dementia and found that six fulfilled their designated inclusion criteria. Taking age and sex into consideration they could find no major geographical differences in the prevalence of Alzheimer's disease between the European studies, and found overall percentages for prevalence between the ages of 30–59 of 0.02%; 60–69, 0.3%; 70–79, 3.1%; and 80–89, 10.8% (Rocca *et al.*, 1991). They comment that prevalence increased exponentially with advancing age and that in some populations it was consistently higher in women.

Rorsman *et al.* (1986) reported the results of their longitudinal study of prevalence and incidence in the island of Lundby, which started in 1947 and ended in 1972. At first they reported a decline in both senile and multi-infarct dementia over 25 years. However, when those who entered the study in 1957 were added to the sample no significant difference over time was found. For the incidence rates for 1947–1957 and 1957–1972, respectively, they derived figures of 6.7 and 4.9 per 1000 men per year and 8.4 and 5.2 per 1000 women. Dartigues *et al.* (quoted by Launer *et al.*, 1992) have also reported incidence rates for dementia from their Bordeaux study. The overall incidence is 11 persons per 1000 per year.

Studies are now being undertaken using the same standardized methods of data collection and a computer assisted, and therefore consistent, method of diagnosis. Copeland *et al.* (1987a) reported the first comparative study using the GMS–AGECAT package (Copeland *et al.*, 1986; Dewey and

Copeland, 1986) to compare populations in New York and London. Almost twice the level of dementia was found in New York compared with London. This increase was found for every half decade of life after the age of 65 and for five out of the six separately drawn random samples. The cases of dementia were clinically confirmed by follow-up one year later. Most of the obvious possible causes for the differences in prevalence were thought to have been excluded. This finding remains the one major difference between geographical areas where the same study methods were used and therefore requires replication. Studies in Liverpool and in an adjacent rural community using similar methods (Copeland *et al.*, 1987b) yielded 4.3% and 3.8%, respectively, for dementia confirmed clinically by follow-up three years later; close to the London figures. A recent, much larger study supported by the Medical Research Council of 5222 subjects in Liverpool yielded a preliminary figure for organic disorders (mostly dementia) of 4.6%, thus demonstrating a satisfactory degree of consistency (Saunders *et al.*, 1993).

Study subjects in Liverpool who had been designated as having mild organic disorder below 'case level' had mainly either recovered or died three years later. Only a small proportion had gone on to develop dementia. Using the same standardized methods, the level for Alzheimer's disease in Liverpool was assessed at 3.3%, that for vascular dementia at 0.7%, and for alcohol related dementia at 0.3%. It will be seen from these studies that the prevalence for dementia and probably also for Alzheimer's disease does not appear to vary between different localities within the UK. The Liverpool group has now followed up its first sample for a number of years and has provided incidence rates for dementia in those aged 65 and over of 9.2 cases of dementia per 1000 of the population per year (Copeland *et al.*, 1992). The corresponding rates are 6.2 for Alzheimer's disease, 2.0 for vascular dementia, and 1.0 per alcohol related dementia. Although these figures appear to differ from those reported above from Bordeaux, if the subjects from both studies are divided into Alzheimer's disease, vascular dementia and others, the rate for Alzheimer's disease is remarkably close in the two studies and the difference lies almost entirely in the category of 'other' which achieves a higher level in Bordeaux. It would appear that incidence figures for dementia are beginning to agree at around 1% per year.

The MRC–ALPHA study of 5222 subjects in Liverpool which had an age stratified sample, showed clearly that the levels of dementia rise consistently throughout the age span well into the tenth decade (Saunders *et al.*, 1993).

Numerous studies of the prevalence of dementia have been undertaken in other parts of the world but are difficult to interpret because of the problem of differing methods and definitions. However, some have been undertaken recently using the GMS–AGECAT package and their results are now becoming available. Levels of dementia in Zaragoza in Spain of 7.5%, although apparently high are not significantly different from those in Liverpool (Lobo *et al.*, 1992). The only figures so far provided by the Pan American Health Organization studies in Latin America are for Santiago, Chile at 4.6%. Kua (1991) found 2.3% of dementia in the Chinese community of Singapore before adjusting the age of the population for comparison with that of Liverpool. Using the GMS but with a psychiatrist's diagnosis Kua found a figure of 1.8%, identical to that found by Li *et al.* (1989) in Beijing using the GMS, but not the computer diagnosis AGECAT. Kay *et al.* (1985) in Hobart, Tasmania found 7.7% in subjects aged 70 and over using the GMS–AGECAT system compared with 7.3% for that age group in Liverpool. Engedal *et al.* (1988) found 10.8% using the GMS without the AGECAT diagnosis in Norway for subjects aged 75 and over, showing remarkably similar figures to the 10.5% found in Liverpool for this age group. Using standardized methods for comparative studies between the UK and countries abroad can reveal very similar figures for dementia as a whole. Earlier studies in Japan (Hasegawa *et al.*, 1986) quoted higher figures for vascular dementia than for dementia of the Alzheimer type. More recent studies have tended to show levels of vascular disorder which have not been so high but which still account for more than half the dementias found. It is possible that the lower levels of Alzheimer's disease previously quoted in these studies may have arisen, once again due to the use of different methods and definitions. However, these matters need further evaluation. A large study by Zhang *et al.* (1990) in Shanghai using the Mini-Mental State Examination (Folstein *et al.*, 1975) modified for cultural factors gave an overall figure for dementia of 4.6% for persons aged 55 and over.

Jorm *et al.* (1987) reviewing studies published between 1945 and 1985 came to the conclusion that the prevalence of dementia in subjects aged over 65 roughly doubled for each half decade of life. Again, this meta-analysis did not find a difference in the levels for men and women. The MRC–ALPHA study in Liverpool which forms part of the Multi-site Study of Cognitive Function and Ageing in the UK shows a clear preponderance of women with dementia except in the 65–79 age bracket.

The problem of the mild dementias has been mentioned above. It has been further explored by O'Connor *et al.* (1991) who found no sharp boundaries between findings for older people with no dementia, and those with minimal and mild dementia as assessed by ratings of disability and memory. They point out the importance of confounding factors such as drug and other forms of intoxication, and deafness which produce minor errors in assessment. An interview with an informant is usually regarded as important for clinical work but such an interview has often been omitted from epidemiological studies. It may however, prove essential for resolving the presence of dementia in certain cases. The principal standardized methods now contain informant interviews and Jorm *et al.* (1991) reported a useful method, the

'IQ CODE', for obtaining valuable information from an informant if the patient is unable to respond to the examination appropriately.

CAUSAL AND RISK FACTORS

The search for causal and risk factors for Alzheimer's disease and the other dementias continues. Age and positive family history for dementia are the two principal risk factors so far identified. Suffering from Down's syndrome seems, in many cases, to predispose to dementia later in life. Some, but not all, studies have shown a clear preponderance of women with dementia. Genetic factors must certainly play a part in the causation of the Alzheimer's disease commonly found in clinical practice, but they appear to play an even greater role in the familial types which are comparatively rare. The reanalyses of studies examining the role of head injury preceding sporadic dementia now seem to show that this risk factor is standing up to rigorous testing (Mortimer *et al.*, 1991). Other putative risk factors under examination are past history of hypothyroidism, depressive illness (late onset), exposure to aluminium and lead, and maternal ages of 15–19 years and over 40 years. Recently, Hebert *et al.* (1992), working in East Boston on community subjects, found that the risk for Alzheimer's disease in their longitudinal studies was associated with up to seven years of schooling compared with those with more substantial education. They found neither alcohol consumption nor tobacco smoking to be associated with risk. Earlier, Graves *et al.* (1991) had postulated an inverse relationship between dementia and a history of tobacco smoking. In the Liverpool studies, Saunders *et al.* (1991) also using concurrent prospective methods found that a period of heavy drinking of at least five years at some time in the subject's life was associated with a five-fold increased risk of dementia in elderly men although they were not necessarily drinking at the time of examination. Because of the different methods and case definitions used it is still not possible to be sure that differences found for risk factors are other than artefacts of these methods.

The similar results for the levels of dementia and Alzheimer's disease in different parts of the world, although disappointing to the epidemiologist searching for risk factors, do raise interesting questions as to how a disease with both genetic and environmental components could emerge with such similar levels in such diverse geographical and racially different areas.

IMPLICATIONS FOR THE FUTURE

All studies show the steep rise in both the prevalence and incidence of dementia as a whole and of Alzheimer's disease in particular with age. Yet it is just those older age groups of the population in which Alzheimer's disease is most common, which are set to grow in proportion until well into the next century. The tendency has been for forecasts of population change to underestimate growth, so Alzheimer's disease must be expected to present a serious and costly problem to the providers of health care for the future. So much will depend on adequate community resources to sustain victims of the disease for as long as possible outside residential care. But will sufficient women, who still make up the majority of informal and formal carers still be available to keep up with need. Changing educational patterns and employment prospects, increasing independence, the break up of family units and increased mobility may all limit the availability of such a cheap, if effective, provision of care. The proportion of ill older people living alone and potentially requiring a greater concentration of service help continues to grow. The outcome of such factors is always difficult to predict and everything could change dramatically if medication were discovered which substantially improved or arrested the progress of the disease.

REFERENCES

American Psychiatric Association (1980). *Diagnostic and Statistical Manual of Mental Disorders (DSM III) 3rd edn.* American Psychiatric Association, Washington, DC.

Bondareff W. (1983). Age and Alzheimer's disease. *Lancet,* **ii**, 1447.

Clarke, M., Lowry, R. and Clarke, S. (1986). Cognitive impairment in the elderly—a community survey. *Age Ageing*, **15**, 278–284.

Copeland, J.R.M., Dewey, M.E. and Griffiths-Jones, H.M. (1986). Computerised psychiatric diagnosis system and case nomenclature for elderly subjects: GMS and AGECAT. *Psychol. Med.*, **16**, 89–99.

Copeland, J.R.M., Gurland, B.J., Dewey, M.E., Kelleher, M.J., Smith, A.M.R. and Davidson, I.A. (1987a). Is there more dementia, depression and neurosis in New York? A comparative community study of the elderly in New York and London using the computer diagnosis, AGECAT. *Br. J. Psychiatry*, **151**, 466–473.

Copeland, J.R.M., Dewey, M.E., Wood, N., Searle, R., Davidson, I.A. and McWilliam, C. (1987b). The range of mental illness amongst the elderly in the community: prevalence in Liverpool. *Br. J. Psychiatry*, **150**, 815–823.

Copeland, J.R.M., Davidson, I.A., Dewey, M.E., Gilmore, C., Larkin, B.A., McWilliam, C., Saunders, P.A., Scott, A., Sharma, V. and Sullivan, C. (1992). Alzheimer's disease, other dementias, depression and pseudodementia: prevalence, incidence and three-year outcome in Liverpool. *Br. J. Psychiatry*, **161**, 230–239.

Dewey, M.E. and Copeland, J.R.M. (1986). Computerised psychiatric diagnosis in the elderly: AGECAT. *J. Microcomp. Appl.*, **9**, 135–140.

Engedal, K., Gilke, K. and Laake, K. (1988). Prevalence of dementia in a Norwegian sample aged 75 years and older and living at home. *Comp. Gerontol. A*, **2**, 102–106.

Folstein, M.F., Folstein, S.E. and McHugh, P.R. (1975). Mini-mental state: a practical method for grading the cognitive state of patients for the clinician. *J. Psychiatr. Res.*, **12**, 189–198.

Graves, A.B., Van Duijn, C.M., Chandra, V., Fratiglioni, I., Heyman, A., Jorm, A.F., Kokmen, E., Kondo, K., Mortimer, J.A., Rocca, W.A., Shalat, S.I., Soininen, H. and Hofman, A. for the EURODEM Risk Factors Research Group (1991). Alcohol and tobacco consumption as risk factors for Alzheimer's disease: a collaborative re-analysis of case control studies. *Int. J. Epidemiol.*, **20** (Suppl 2), 48–57.

Hasegawa, K., Homma, A. and Imai, Y. (1986). An epidemiological study of age related dementia in the community. *Int. J. Geriatr. Psychiatry*, **1**, 45–55.

Hebert, L.E., Scherr, P.A., Beckett, L.A., Funkenstein, H.H., Albert, M.S., Chown, M.J. and Evans, D.A. (1992). Relation of smoking and alcohol consumption to incident Alzheimer's disease. *Am. J. Epidemiol.*, **135**, 347–355.

Jagger, C., Clarke, M., Anderson, J. and Battcock, T. (1992). Dementia in Melton Mowbray—a validation of earlier findings. *Age Ageing*, **21**, 205–210.

Jorm, A.F., Korten, A.E. and Henderson, A.S. (1987). The prevalence of dementia: a quantitative integration of the literature. *Acta Psychiatr. Scand.*, **76**, 465–479.

Jorm, A.F., Scott, R., Cullen, J.S. and MacKinnon, A.J. (1991). Performance of the informant questionnaire on cognitive decline in the elderly (IQ CODE) as a screening test for dementia. *Psychol. Med.*, **21**, 785–790.

Kay, D.W.K. (1991). The epidemiology of dementia: a review of recent work. *Rev. Clin. Gerontol.*, **1**, 55–66.

Kay, D.W.K., Beamish, R. and Roth, M. (1964). Old age mental disorders in Newcastle upon Tyne. Part I. A study of prevalence. *Br. J. Psychiatry*, **110**, 146–158.

Kay, D.W.K., Henderson, A.S., Scott, R., Wilson, J., Rickwood, D. and Grayson, D.A. (1985). Dementia and depression among the elderly living in the Hobart community: the effect of the diagnostic criteria on the prevalence rates. *Psychol. Med.*, **15**, 771–788.

Kokmen, E., Beard, M., Offord, K.P. and Kurland, L.T. (1989). Prevalence of medically diagnosed dementia in a defined United States population: Rochester, Minnesota. *Neurology*, **39**, 773–775.

Kua, E.H. (1991). The prevalence of dementia in elderly chinese. *Acta Psychiatr. Scand.*, **83**, 350–352.

Launer, L.J., Brayne, C., Dartigues, J.-F. and Hofman, A. (1992). Epilogue. *Neuroepidemiology*, **11** (Suppl. 1), 119–121.

Li, G., Shen, Y.C., Chen, C.H., Zhao, Y.W., Li, S.R. and Lu, M. (1989). An epidemiological survey of age-related dementia in an urban area of Beijing. *Acta Psychiatr. Scand.*, **79**, 557–563.

Livingstone, G., Hawkins, A., Graham, N., Blizard, R. and Mann, A.H. (1990). The Gospel Oak Study: prevalence rates of dementia depression and activity limitation among elderly residents in inner London. *Psychol. Med.*, **20**, 137–146.

Lobo, A., Dewey, M.E., Copeland, J.R.M., Dia, J.L. and Saz, P. (1992). The prevalence of dementia in the community elderly of Zaragoza and Liverpool: a preliminary communication. *Psychol. Med.*, **22**, 239–243.

McKeith, I., Fairbairn, A., Perry, R., Thompson, P. and Perre, E. (1992). Neuroleptic sensitivity in patients with senile dementia of Lewy body type. *Br. Med. J.*, **305**, 673–678.

McKhann, G., Drachman, D., Folstein, M., Katzman, R., Price, D. and Stadlan, E.M. (1984). Clinical diagnosis of Alzheimer's disease: report of the NINCDS–ADRDA Work Group under the auspices of Department of Health and Human Services Task Force on Alzheimer's Disease. *Neurology*, **34**, 939–944.

Molsa, P.K., Marttila, R.J. and Rinne, U.K. (1982). Epidemiology of dementia in a Finnish population. *Acta Neurol. Scand.*, **65**, 541–552.

Morgan, K., Dalloso, H.M., Arie, T., Bryne, E.J., Jones, R. and Waite, J. (1987). Mental health and psychological well-being among the old and very old living at home. *Br. J. Psychiatry*, **150**, 808–814.

Mortimer, J.A., Duijn, C.M., Chandra, V., Fratiglioni, L., Graves, A.B., Heyman, A., Jorm, A.F., Kokmen, E., Kondo, K., Rocca, W.A., Shalat, S.L., Soininen, H. and Hofman, A. (1991). For the EURODEM risk factors research group. Head trauma as a risk factor for Alzheimer's disease: a collaborative re-analysis of case control studies. *Int. J. Epidemiol*, **20** (Suppl. 2), 62–64.

O'Connor, D.W., Pollitt, P.A., Hyde, J.B., Fellowes, J.L., Miller, N.D., Brook, C.P.B., Reiss, R.B. and Roth, M. (1989). The prevalence of dementia as measured by the Cambridge Mental Disorders of the Elderly Examination. *Acta Psychiatr. Scand.*, **79**, 190–198.

O'Connor, D.W., Pollitt, P.A., Hyde, J.B., Miller, N.D. and Fellowes, J.L. (1991). Clinical issues relating to the diagnosis of mild dementia in a British community survey (1991). *Arch. Neurol.*, **48**, 530–534.

Robertson, D., Rockwood, K. and Stolee, P. (1989). The prevalence of cognitive impairment in an elderly Canadian population. *Acta Psychiatr. Scand.*, **80**, 303–309.

Rocca, W.A., Hofman, A., Brayne, C., Breteler, M., Clarke, M., Copeland, J.R.M., Dartigues, J.F., Engedal, K., Hagnell, O., Heeren, T.J., Jonker, C., Lindesay, J., Lobo, A., Mann, A.H., Morgan, K., O'Connor, D.W., Da Silvaproux, A., Sulkava, R., Kay, D.W.K. and Amaducci, L. (1991). Frequency and distribution of Alzheimer's disease in Europe: collaborative study of 1980–1990 prevalence findings. *Ann. Neurol.*, **30**, 381–390.

Rorsman, B., Hagnell, O. and Lanke, J. (1986). Prevalence and incidence of senile and multi-infarct dementia in the Lundby study: a comparison between the time periods 1947–1957 and 1957–1972. *Neuropsychobiology*, **15**, 122–129.

Roth, M., Tym, E., Mountjoy, C.Q., Huppert, F.A., Hendrie, H., Verma, S. and Goddard, R. (1986). CAMDEX. A standardised instrument for the diagnosis of mental disorders in the elderly with special reference to the early detection of dementia. *Br. J. Psychiatry*, **149**, 698–709.

Saunders, P.A., Copeland, J.R.M., Dewey, M.E., Davidson, I.A., McWilliam, C., Sharma, V. and Sullivan, C. (1991). Heavy drinking as a risk factor for depression and dementia in elderly men: findings from the Liverpool Longitudinal Community Study. *Br. J. Psychiatry*, **159**, 213–216.

Saunders, P.A., Copeland, J.R.M., Dewey, M.E., Gilmore, C., Larkin, B.A., Phaterpekar, H. and Scott, A. (1993). The prevalence of dementia, depression and neurosis in later life: findings from the Liverpool MRC-ALPHA study. *Int. J. Epidemiol.*, in press.

Sulkava, R., Wikstrom, J., Aromaa, A., Raitasalo, R., Lehtinen, V., Lahtela, K. and Palo, J. (1985). Prevalence of severe dementia in Finland. *Neurology*, **35**, 1025–1029.

Zhang, M., Katzman, R., Salmon, D., Jin, H., Cai, G., Wang, Z., Qu, G., Grant, I., Yu, E., Levy, P., Klaber, M.R. and Liu, W. (1990). The prevalence of dementia and Alzheimer's disease in Shanghai, China; impact of age, gender, and education. *Ann. Neurol.*, **27**, 428–437.

2

Resource and Government: The Political Context of Alzheimer's Disease

THOMAS K.B. DELANEY

Magellan Medical Communications Ltd, London, UK

INTRODUCTION

[handwritten: Lil renè carers – unpaid]

The seventeenth annual symposium of the Texas Records Institute of Mental Services was held 23–26 October 1983 in Houston, Texas; its title was 'Aging 2000: Our Health Care Destiny'. As others in the current volume describe, Alzheimer's disease (AD) is destiny for some of us. Indeed, the bell will toll, as it already has for many millions whose dignity and personality have been taken from them, leaving only the silhouette of someone who, in earlier days, was a contributor to social and family life. The problem is that the silhouette still casts a long shadow. AD is no respecter of social, family or intellectual status; it reaches victims from the top to the bottom of our everyday life, from the rich, famous and influential to the man on the Clapham omnibus.

AD has a fundamental feature which distinguishes it from other major age-related illnesses—it reaches the entire fabric of family life, and as the disease progresses it places a sometimes intolerable stress on the 'carer'. The role of the carer in AD is unparalleled in medicine. The sufferer can be fit and strong, sometimes too fit and strong, but we know they are deprived of many of the intellectual processes that form personality and the power of rational thought and the ability to converse in a non-repetitive fashion. This knowledge is of little comfort to the carer who is unrecognized, and love becomes a one-sided emotion.

AD has been described many times, we know the misery and suffering it causes, we are aware of the feeble attempts at treatment and of the great competition amongst the scientific community and the pharmaceutical industry to begin the therapeutic process. Indeed, by the time of publication it is hoped that a compound, whilst not a cure, but the first in a long line of evolving compounds that will end the misery that is AD, will be with us.

The first step in the psysician's therapeutic armamentarium will only serve to focus attention on the roulette wheel of the dementia.

The first therapeutic agent will doubtless highlight the misery of those it cannot help and so expose the burden this disease imposes upon the patient, carer, society, health care professional and central government. This one disease has the potential to bring the National Health Service to its knees, a service that despite its many critics is widely regarded as the finest system of health care in the world.

THE SOCIAL PROBLEM

The profound growth of the elderly population is undeniable. The last 40 years have seen substantial increases of those aged 65 years and over. Currently, the elderly represent almost 16% of the UK population. Of particular concern to health care providers is the expansion of the very elderly, those aged 75–85, and it is the projected growth of this group that is the most worrying.

Figure 1 shows the rapid rise of the 75–85 age group over the past five decades. Demographic ageing is a consequence of falling birth rates and increasing life expectancy, the latter being a triumph of modern day medicine.

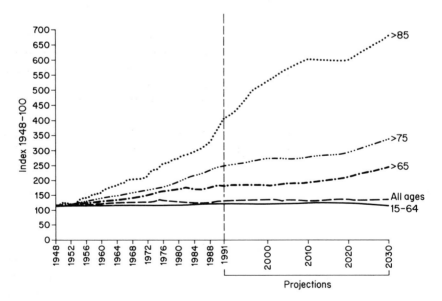

Figure 1. The rapid rise of the 75–85 age group over the past five decades.

Table 1. The annual resource cost of all health and social services to people aged 65+ with Alzheimer's Disease, England 1990/91 (£ millions).

Item	Age-groups			Percent
	65–74	75+	Total	
Acute/geriatric hospital in-patient care	4.365	72.091	76.456	7.3
Acute/geriatric hospital out-patient care	0.057	0.513	0.569	0.05
Mental hospital in- and out-patient care	29.720	155.985	185.705	17.9
General practice consultations	0.423	3.305	3.728	0.4
Residential care in:				
Private residential homes	6.791	248.186	254.978	24.6
Voluntary residential homes	1.607	58.646	60.253	5.8
Local authority accommodation	6.568	239.610	246.178	23.7
Private/voluntary nursing homes	3.056	111.725	114.780	11.0
Day/care (local authority and other providers)	0.825	2.776	3.601	0.3
Home care	6.079	19.958	26.038	2.5
Informal care payment (AA and ICA)	4.371	60.629	65.000	6.3
Total	**63.862**	**973.424**	**1037.286**	**100**
Percent	**6.2**	**93.8**	**100**	

Source: Adapted from Fenn and Gray (1993).

The elderly, particularly those in the 75–85 age group, are massive consumers of health care resources. A recent study by Fenn and Gray (1993) estimated that costs of AD in England alone were in excess of £1 billion (£1000 million) per annum.

Table 1 shows the distribution of resource costs of AD by type of care and provider. It clearly demonstrates that the 75+ age group consume the vast majority of scarce health care resources. This figure makes no allowance for the cost to the carer. A study by Hay and Ernst in 1987 estimated an annual US cost of $28–31 billion. Given that this is the age group that is the fastest growing and that AD is age-related, we have the principal reason for concern amongst so many of the world's health care providers.

The cost of looking after a person with AD is so burdensome that, in the United States, a phenomenon known as 'granny dumping' has occurred. Whilst this may seem abhorrent to those of us who have not cared for someone with AD, it could be argued that the end stage AD patient, incontinent of faeces and urine, unable to recognize loved ones, disorientated in space and time, a major strain upon family life and potentially leading to its break-up, really does not mind. As the fate of the AD sufferer becomes known, so does the existence of 'living wills', now legal in some parts of Europe—a very real and provocative challenge to society.

It is the duty of all members of society, young and old, to establish a powerful lobby group that specifically has input into the design of 'policy' vis-à-vis care of the elderly. In particular, it must ensure that in these days of ever increasing budgetary control, that 'high cost' conditions such as AD are not discriminated against. The role, purpose and value of the carer *must* also be recognized. Adequate resource should be given; there is enormous scope for improvement.

THE POLITICAL CHALLENGE

By the year 2000, the world's population of elderly will be approaching 600 million. An ageing population is now unique to the UK. Every major developed country of the OCED is experiencing a rapid expansion of its elderly population. The UK, however, does have one of the highest ratios of elderly people (65 years and over) to population. Table 2 shows elderly persons (male and female) as a percentage of the total UK population.

In many countries, no coherent approach to the 'quiet epidemic' is in evidence. The *British Medical Journal* carried a leading article in 1978 warning us of the advancing tide of the elderly, mentally infirm. As Arie (1984) has pointed out, the epidemic is so vast 'that it is often unnoticed'.

Certainly, Government ministers have been remarkably reluctant to invest in AD in the same way as in other, perhaps more fashionable, areas of research. This is not to say that funding is totally absent. All European Governments have some AD research, and in the UK the Alzheimer's Disease Society receives some £130 000 per annum from The Department of Health to assist in its aims and objectives.

The EC has rather more ambitious plans to stimulate neurological research and has named the 1990s as a 'European Decade of Brain Research'. In support of this a document has been produced, Report A3–0222/92, which was published 18 June 1992. It focuses especially on AD and highlights the very real cost of neurological disease. Perhaps it will generate as much research as President Kennedy's 'we shall have a man on the moon by the end of the

Table 2. Elderly persons as percentage of UK total population (males & females).

	>65	>75	75–84	>85
1948	10.7%	3.4%	3.0%	0.4%
1950	10.7%	3.6%	3.1%	0.5%
1960	11.7%	4.2%	3.6%	0.6%
1970	13.0%	4.6%	3.8%	0.8%
1980	14.9%	5.7%	4.6%	1.0%
1990	15.6%	6.9%	5.4%	1.5%
2001[a]	15.5%	7.4%	5.5%	1.9%
2011[a]	16.1%	7.4%	5.3%	2.1%
2021[a]	17.9%	7.9%	5.8%	2.1%
2031[a]	20.4%	9.1%	6.8%	2.3%

[a]Projections based on 1989 mid-year estimates.
Source: OPCS (1991)

decade' pronouncement. It is noteworthy that the report recognizes that research will find a cure for AD, but it remains questionable whether or not it is providing a suitable base for academic and industrial research to find a 'cure' by the end of the decade. Whether it is a fear of the rising health care costs of the elderly or true pragmatism that is driving our research goals, it is clear that we need to restructure our present research priorities, to revalue the profound contemporary dilemma of the 'greying' of nations.

To do this we must immediately amend our current financing and organization of research, encourage and adapt report A3–0222/92, and Government must perform its duty to the electorate and direct and motivate research, not merely to find a cure for AD or even to extend life, but to extend the vigorous and productive years. To do this would be a major political achievement, it would also be self-financing, as more and more of us become classified as elderly and continue to make positive contributions to society.

The elderly need a political champion, not one approaching elevation to the House of Lords. We need a politician with compassion and vision, to put aside party politics and to look forward perhaps 25 years, to set in motion a period of research that will end in a cure, rather than the staccato movement of every four or five years in office. As Archimedes said 'Give me somewhere to stand, and I will move the earth'; perhaps this is what political union really should be about.

CONCLUSION

As Busse commented almost a decade ago, at the seventeenth annual symposium of the Texas Research Institute of Mental Sciences 'the allocation of limited resources will be a serious problem for the medical profession and will be a major political issue'. Unless, in this the European Year of the Elderly, Government truly grasps the consequences of the 'greying' of nations, it is unlikely that the sunset years of life will be ones we can look forward to with optimism.

Comes a time
When even the old and familiar ideas
Float out of reach of the mind's hooks
And the soul's prime
Has slipped like a fish through the once high weirs
Of an ailing confidence. O where are the books
On this kind of death?

(From: Desmond O'Grady, 'The Poet in Old Age Fishing at Evening' for Ezra Pound.)

REFERENCES

Arie, T. (1984). Senile dementia: outlook for the future. In: Wertheimer, J. and Marois, M. (Eds), *Senile Dementia*. Liss, New York, pp. 201–209.

British Medical Journal (1978). The quiet epidemic (leading article). *Br. Med. J.*, **1**, 1.

Fenn, P. and Gray, A. (1993). Alzheimer's Disease: the burden of illness in England. *Health Trends*, **25**, 1.

Hay, J.W. and Ernst, R.L. (1987). The economic costs of Alzheimer's Disease. *Am. J. Pub. Health*, **77**, 1169–1175.

OPCS (Office of Population Censuses and Surveys) (1991). *General Household Survey 1989*, (Series GHS No. 20). HMSO, London.

Royal College of General Practitioners, Department of Health and Social Security, Office of Population Censuses and Surveys (1986). *Morbidity Statistics from General Practice: 3rd National Study 1981–82*, (Series MBS No. 1). HMSO, London.

II

Assessment and Diagnosis

3

Practical Aspects of Diagnosis and Early Recognition of Alzheimer's Disease

PAUL R. GROB

Professor of General Practice and Health Care Research, Robens Institute, University of Surrey, Guildford, UK

INTRODUCTION

Old age, especially when the alternative is considered, is becoming increasingly popular.

At the turn of the century the average life expectancy was 49, now it is in the upper 70s. In 1980, 12% of the population was over 65 years, by 2030 this will increase to 22%. At higher age ranges the increase is greater with the number of over 80s projecting to more than double from 2.1% to 5% of the total population from the years 1980–2030 (OCED, 1987).

The incidence of dementia is high, affecting up to 16% of the over 65s and escalating to 36% of the over 80s (Pfeffer *et al.*, 1987; Clarke *et al.*, 1991). At present 50 million people world-wide suffer from dementia and the number of dementia cases is estimated to rise by 50% by the year 2050. Future financial implications of providing care for the dementing elderly are not insignificant, the projected cost of medication by the year 2000 will be $3 million (Moran, 1991). The average projected increase in total health expenditure is 30% over the next 50 years of which 20% would be used in the care of the elderly (OCED, 1987). This is an average figure, for countries such as Japan and Canada these increases will be far higher as a greater proportion of the population will be elderly (OCED, 1987; see also Copeland, Chapter 1, and Delaney, Chapter 2, this volume).

In addition, much effort is directed at increasing lifespan by active intervention. However, there is little point in doing this if the extra years are spent struggling with mental or physical disability.

European data suggest that advances in reducing mortality have been accompanied by slower progress in reducing morbidity. People live longer but have to put up with disability for longer, too. Over the 10 years between 1976 and 1985 in England the absolute number of years to be lived with disability increased by 1.3 years in men to 13.1 years and by 2.2 years in women to 16.2 years. Broadly comparable data have been reported from France, where women may expect to have 11.7 years of disability and men 8.8 years (WHO, 1989).

Dementia was well described by Professor T. Arie (1983) when he wrote:

'*Dementia in the elderly is a global disruption of personality, affecting behaviour and intelligence, with impairment of the ability to learn new responses, and thus to adapt to a changing environment. The emotional response is disorganized and blunted, most striking of all there is loss of the ability to remember recent events. Often an astonishing degree of function may be preserved, provided the person retains a constant environment with which he/she is familiar and that new demands on him/her are not great. Even so, such preservation is always precarious, depending on a constancy and security which are unlikely to last long.*'

DEMENTIA—THE GENERAL CLINICAL PICTURE

There are several presenting clinical features of dementia associated with the impairment of memory, intellect and personality.

Memory

Classically memory for recent events is lost first. The patient can remember events, names and places from earlier years, but recent memory may be lost. In addition Alzheimer's sufferers may notice memory loss as the first symptom they themselves observe. They may take note of things to do as a checklist, but memory loss especially in patients with a high intellectual capacity may be very distressing indeed. The inability to go shopping and handle money is often what alerts the sufferer and his family to the possibility of a serious condition.

Intellect

Intellectual impairment is characterized by the inability to cope with new situations, to separate important things from trivia and to grasp facts. False ideas and delusions may also be present and care should be taken if it is the sufferer who normally handles the family finances and investments to ensure that help is provided to avoid catastrophic financial decisions.

Personality changes

Perhaps the most devastating changes are those associated with a deterioration of personality. The patient may become a caricature of features previously held in check. This may result in meanness, tactlessness, impulsiveness, laziness, over-concern with health and sexual perversion. Eventually the whole personality may change. The sufferer will have 'good' and 'bad' days for no apparent reason: there may be a phase in which extremes of behaviour and 'being difficult' are very common; however, as the disease progresses this may give way to a much more benign and easy to handle childlike personality. Eventually the sufferer may appear to lose touch with his carer and loved ones and appear to have little or no reaction to people or his surroundings.

There may also be an increasing preoccupation with self and a narrowing of interest, for example, the patient may cease to go to the theatre or to football matches.

Intolerance of change

Intolerance of change is common and this may be seen in many people who would not regard themselves as demented. The person may be querulous and sometimes explode, becoming irritable and agitated before collapsing into tearful helplessness.

Depression

Depression is also a feature of dementia, occurring in about 25% of patients and it is important that its presence is noted since it may respond to antidepressant therapy. Depression in dementia is variable. There may be self-deprecating, accusing, bizarre or extravagant delusions.

It is not unusual for the elderly demented patient to accuse his relatives or the staff who are helping him of things which they have not done. The depression may be interrupted by episodes of clouding of consciousness or amnesia. Serious suicide attempts may be made during an episode of clouding.

Spatial orientation

Another fundamental change in dementia is the disturbance of cortical functions. There may be disturbance of spatial orientation and body image with aphasia and apraxia. Patients may lose their way in familiar surroundings or show unexplained lapses in long-established skills. These changes may sometimes occur before there is significant impairment of memory or intellect.

Delirium

In dementia caused by organic disease, there may be clouded or delirious states caused by the underlying disease.

DIFFERENTIAL DIAGNOSIS

One important factor, if improvement by therapy is desired, is to be able to distinguish the most common types of dementia and to recognize their characteristic features so diagnosis can be made at an early stage.

In Alzheimer's disease there is a progressive and seemingly relentless deterioration of memory, intellect and personality. There is a blunting of emotions, a reduction of initiative and a loss of insight as the patient seems unaware of the memory impairment. Associated with these factors is a gradually progressive decrease in physical strength.

In multi-infarct, *non-Alzheimer type*, dementia associated with underlying organic disease, there is also a deterioration of memory, intellect and personality but it is *not* relentless. There is emotional incontinence but insight is preserved. The patient is aware of memory impairment and often makes an excuse. For example, when asked what day it is, the patient may say: 'I've not seen the paper today'. This type of dementia is not progressive in the same way as is Alzheimer's disease; it has a remittent and fluctuating course. Alzheimer's disease rarely, if ever, responds to treatment, where dementia associated with organic disease may well respond.

Thus dementia can usefully be sub-classified, e.g. into senile dementia of Alzheimer type (SDAT) and the less common multi-infarct dementia (MID). Clinically they may be distinguished; an abrupt onset with a step-wise, fluctuating course and the presence of focal neurological signs favours a diagnosis

Table 1. The Hachinski Scale.

Clinical feature	Score
Abrupt onset	2
Step-wise deterioration	1
Fluctuating course	2
Nocturnal confusion	1
Relative preservation of personality	1
Depression	1
Somatic complaints	1
Emotional incontinence	1
History of hypertension	1
History of strokes	2
Evidence of associated atherosclerosis	1
Focal neurological symptoms	2
Focal neurological signs	2

of MID. A useful scoring system devised by Hachinski (1975) gives some guidance to the likelihood of a patient suffering from MID, the higher the score on the Hachinski scale the greater the probability of MID (Table 1). Recently it has become clear that senile dementia of Lewy body type (SDLT) must also be considered carefully as it probably occurs more frequently than previously suspected.

History and clinical examination

Early diagnosis is important if patients suffering from dementia and their carers are to be successfully helped. The condition is often missed because some doctors regard it as normal for elderly people to become forgetful.

We do all become a little forgetful, but when it is more than a little forgetful, we should take notice and look into the problem. If a patient makes repeated obvious mistakes like forgetting to put milk bottles out, forgetting to wash or dress properly, then further investigation is warranted.

A good history and clinical examination are essential so that any physical illness which may be promoting or enhancing the patient's mental state can be recognized and treated. Thus, before a definite diagnosis of dementia is made alternative conditions should be excluded, these include a toxic confusional state, potentially reversible intracranial lesions, depression and psychotic illness.

Toxic confusional state is often caused by infection, especially respiratory or urinary, current medication, excess alcohol, or head injury. Generalized medical conditions like carcinomatosis, cardiac, hepatic or liver failure can all produce the picture of a confused toxic patient.

Depression may mimic dementia in as much as a high proportion of elderly patients with an acute depressive illness show some features similar to dementia, such as memory impairment. A careful history, however, will usually elicit important diagnostic clues; a previous personality history of depression together with the fact that the depressive symptoms preceded intellectual impairment point to this diagnosis. However, clinical experience suggests that a trial of one of the newer antidepressants may well be worthwhile to see if it results in clinical improvement.

Diet should be investigated; elderly patients often take a diet deficient in potassium, and studies have shown evidence of potassium deficiency in depressive and demented patients. Some patients especially if they wander continually require a high calorific input simply to maintain their body weight.

TREATMENT OF DEMENTIA IN THE COMMUNITY SETTING

The practising clinician faces a difficult dilemma in the treatment of senile dementia in the community. 'Nothing can be done, it's her age' is not exactly helpful and leaves the carers especially with a sense of isolation and frustration. Conversely, patients can be over-treated by the physician either in the belief that 'there is a cure for every ill' or because there is great pressure from the carers or relatives for tranquillizers or sedatives to be given to the patient to try to ameliorate an increasingly difficult home situation. Polypharmacy is common in the elderly as they tend to accumulate a 'shopping list of drugs', often given over time, by different and well-meaning clinicians. Indeed some patients seem to be made very much worse by the major tranquillizers.

Several groups of drugs have been developed with the hope of improving cerebral function. These include CNS stimulants and cerebral vasodilators. However, despite optimism, these agents have not been shown to improve markedly the mental status of demented patients.

The need for more effective agents in dementia continues and it must be hoped that progress can continue to be made in this extremely difficult field.

A major part of the 'treatment' of the dementing patient is to give the carer information about the disease and its natural history, so that the quality of home care can be maximized. Thus an important role for the treating physician is to ensure that the carer is put in contact with the excellent self help and support groups run by the Alzheimer's Disease Society. The publications *Caring for the Person with Dementia* (Alzheimer's Disease Society, 1991) and *The 36 Hour Day* (Mace *et al.*, 1990) are both excellent and valuable mines of information and sound practical advice on caring for the demented at home.

Naturally enough the first thing people think about with an Alzheimer's patient is the physical side of managing the illness, however as Sacks well remarked 'people do not consist of memory alone. People have feelings, imagination, drive, will and moral being' (Sacks, 1991).

Thus the sufferer deserves to be treated with dignity and respect. Communication should be simple and direct, and eye contact maintained. The attention span may be short so questions should be phrased in such a way as to elicit simple replies: 'Shall we go for a walk today?' is easier to answer than 'What would you like to do today?'. If the person has a religious belief this should be preserved and he should be encouraged to participate in familiar religious ceremonies, as these are often deep rooted and provide a valuable link with earlier normal behaviour.

Safety in the home should be considered, potential hazards like loose rugs, electrical fittings and fires carefully identified and made safe. Many jobs about the house which are traditionally one partner's domain may have to be learnt by the carer.

It is worthwhile to look ahead and seek legal advice so that the family's financial affairs can be managed by the carer or a near relative. It is sometimes prudent to obtain an 'enduring power of attorney' or similar legal document early on in the disease which will greatly simplify financial arrangements in years to come.

Finally, it is vital that carers are encouraged to look after themselves both physically and emotionally. The physical strains of looking after an Alzheimer's sufferer is constant and eroding, the emotional component is equally important. The feelings of anger and guilt should be explored and recognized as normal and common. 'Why me?' is a common feeling at times amongst carers. The Alzheimer's support group plays a vital part in allowing carers to meet with people in a similar predicament, thereby gaining great practical and psychological support.

ASSESSMENT

Mental alertness, disorientation, emotional lability and self care can also be assessed. There have been a number of questionnaires devised to help assess the degree of dementia and whether the patient has improved on treatment. In some cases the effects of treatment are not easily recognized and the use of a standard questionnaire before and after a treatment period helps to distinguish those who have improved, as well as the degree of improvement.

NATURAL HISTORY AND RESEARCH INTO EARLY DEMENTIA

It is important, especially if new drugs are to be tested in dementia, that the natural progression of the disease is understood as fully as possible. Patients entered into drug studies may improve very considerably especially in the first three months of treatment, but this is mainly due to the Hawthorn effect created by the greatly increased attention from doctors and nurses alike when these patients are entered into clinical trials.

For new treatments and therapies to be evaluated properly the natural progression of the disease must be recorded and understood. A large number of psychometric tests have been developed to try to quantify progress in this disease; however, by the nature of the disease the amount of cooperation from the patient may be minimal and their attention span is usually brief. Many tests examine short-term memory and an apparent improvement on a particular psychometric scoring scale may simply be due to the learning effect. Another source of error may be that the very administration of these tests and the associated attention paid to patients if they are in a clinical drug trial may greatly improve their apparent mental ability and health.

A study was undertaken at the University of Surrey (Robinson, personal communication) to evaluate the use of various electrophysiological and psychometric tests in groups of patients presenting with severe memory loss, in order to try to develop reliable objective measuring instruments to assess the decline in patients' suffering from a presumed diagnosis of early dementia. Early in the study it became apparent to health care staff that patients with clear memory defects failed to register as abnormal on either the Mini-Mental State or RCP screening tests, thus the objective of this work was to establish a scale of tests which could be utilized to distinguish and monitor the earliest stages of progressive dementia.

Methods

The study involved assessing the change in memory function in a mixed population of between 60 and 65 years. Subjects were all self-referred and reported suffering from mild to moderate memory problems. Educationally, as a group, they were above the norm which would be expected for this age group (and above the value of our normal group). Initially 56 people were recruited, this dropped to 47 at the second visit and subsequently to 43 willing participants. Testing took place at either the GP's surgery or, where this was not practical, at the Surrey Royal Hospital. A range of psychological and electrophysiological tests were performed three times at approximately six-monthly intervals.

Psychometric tests

The psychometric tests utilized are listed in Table 2 and were administered by the same specially trained research nurse throughout the study.

Table 2. The psychometric tests used in the University of Surrey study.

1. Mini-Mental State examination
2. Yesavage Screen for Dementia
3. RCGP screen for dementia
4. The Graded Naming Test
5. Fuld Object Memory Evaluation
6. The Anomalous Sentence Test
7. Kendrick Cognitive Tests for the Elderly
8. Digit Copying Paradigm
9. Raven Progressive Coloured Matrices
10. Recognition Memory Test, Lexical
11. Benton's Facial Recognition Test

Neurophysiological testing

In order to cross-check any progressive changes seen in the memory loss patients, an objective neurophysiological test was employed.

In this study an endogenous evoked potential, first discovered by Sutton *et al.* (1965), commonly known as the P300 or P3 was used to investigate cortical processing ability in early dementia. By using the P300 it was possible to see not only a response to a stimulus but also a response to conscious thought following recognition of the stimulus.

The exact localization of the P300 component was to some degree irrelevant to this study. The fact that the latency of the P300 had been shown to be delayed in dementia was, however, relevant. Goodin *et al.* (1978) reported on a study of mixed dementias in which he showed 80% had abnormally long P300 latencies. This work had been replicated by Squires *et al.* (1980), Goodin (1986), and Polich (1989) who reported that between 74–80% of their demented patients also showed delayed P300 latency when compared with a normal group. When MIDs and ADs were compared, Polich *et al.* (1987) found little difference in the latency of the delayed P300 when differential diagnosis of early dementias was investigated.

To investigate the use of evoked potential monitoring in old age it was important to have a test which changed little with increasing age. It also had to be reliable and reproducible. Responses had to show definite changes with pathological degeneration and the changes in the early disease stages should be able to be related to other psychological methods. In addition to this, if the test is to be used as a monitoring agent, changes in response should be shown to be a progressive feature running concurrently with other established measures of psychological change.

The P300 test is based on the brain's response to a given stimuli recorded in a similar way to an electroencephalogram with the exception that this test in its simplest form requires only four electrodes and can have an expert system to perform the data analysis.

The simplest form of this test, which is ideal for early screening in dementia, involving presenting the patient with a series of short tones, one of which is at 750 Hz and given for 90% of the presentations within the test. The other which is at 4000 Hz is randomly interspersed within the lower frequency tones. For the test duration the high tone is given a significance. The patient, after first having had a brief preview of the tones, is instructed to quietly count only the high tones. Responses to each type of tone are recorded over the parietal cortex for a period of two seconds following stimulus presentation and are averaged separately to improve signal to noise ratio. The important point to stress at this time is that this response is an endogenous potential, and it is generated within the brain but not by the characteristics of the stimulus.

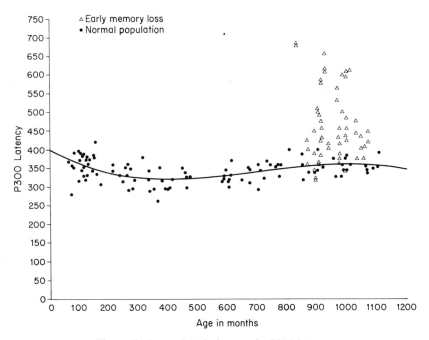

Figure 1. Age related changes in P300 latency.

Results

In the psychometric testing there were no overall significant differences across the three visits. This is partially due to losing the subjects with the most severe memory problems after the first and second visits (this was, in part, due to patients not wishing to have their fears confirmed in the absence of any interventional opportunity) but most significantly due to the remaining people being a mixed population of those showing a definite decline and those remaining the same.

The electrophysiological testing did, however, demonstrate a downward trend during the investigation period. This was exemplified by an increase in the latency of the cognitive evoked potentials. The response latency of the major component of the response, the P3, has been the major feature used in this study.

Figure 1 shows the age related changes in P300 latency in a normal population and in a group of patients with early memory loss.

Subject classification

Thus given the lack of a demonstrable group change in psychometric scores all subjects were examined to see if in there were sub-populations, some of which showed progressive decline.

A method of data investigation, a modification of the sign rank test, marking each change downwards per test and per visit as 1 was employed. This scoring was independent of the actual numerical change except in the case of the P3 data where a threshold of 10 ms was employed. The number of differences found between serial visits and between the first and the last visit were scored and summed for each patient over all the individual psychometric and electrophysiological tests.

Overall there was a large difference between the number of tests per person which declined across the data. Three groups were formed using the psychometric and electrophysiological downward changing scores (DCS).

- Group 1 all showed less than 12 DCS;
- Group 2 were between 13–20 DCS;
- Group 3 had over 20 DCS.

The mean scores for these groups are shown in Figs 2–5. The use of change parameters to classify the subjects' results in a clear separation into three performance groups. Group 1 is different from our normals by 10–15%, whilst group 3 is markedly different across nearly all of the psychometric tests.

Individual subject results

Using the three best tests for showing changes across visits the results for the individual patients are shown by class below. It was of interest to note that not only did the psychometric tests result go down, in some cases they also

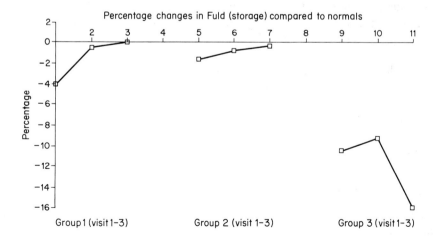

Figure 2. Storage—the ability to 'load' information into memory.

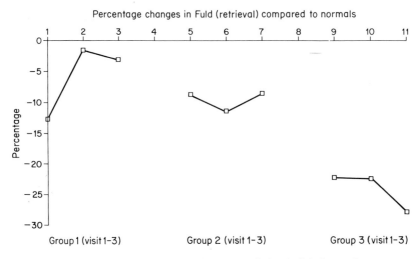

Figure 3. Retrieval—the ability to recall 'loaded' information.

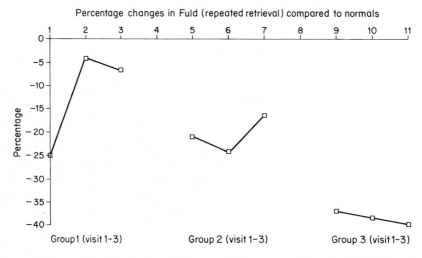

Figure 4. Repeated retrieval—the ability to recall for a second time 'loaded' information.

went up over time. This is well demonstrated in the results for Fuld rapid recall 1 for group 1. Following on from this observation the mean psychometric results from visit 1 to visit 3 were assessed. In group 1, 12 of the individual results improved whilst only one test became worse depicting a strong learning effect. Group 2 improved in six tests but declined in four tests, thus showing a marginal learning effect. Group 3, however, improved

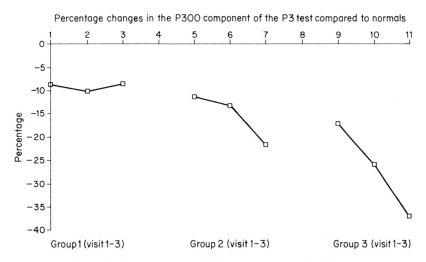

Figure 5. Changes in the P300 component of the P3 test.

in none of the tests and became worse in 14 of them. Thus the population was divided into a mildly affected group, a slightly declining group and a possible pre-dementia group.

Amongst the battery of psychometric tests employed, the Fuld Object Memory Evaluation test was found to be particularly useful. This test is designed specifically for people over 70 years. It involves the feeling and naming of 10 subjects and the subsequent repeated retrieval of their names from memory. This test is initially enjoyable but tends to be rather long so concentration on the part of the more demented patient can begin to wane after the third reminder of forgotten objects. There is more than one form of this test and it would be simple to do three or four forms of it which would eliminate the remembering of previously presented stimuli. In addition to this basic part of the test, distractors are used between each attempt at object recall. These take the form of recall from semantic sets within a set period of time of the number of names, food and vegetables that can be remembered by the patient. The examiner will remind the subject of any of the original objects forgotten after each one of the six trials.

Figures 2–4 show some of the results of this test in the three population groups. Overall the cognitive evoked potentials used on a serial basis offer the most reproducible values in that the test results are not confounded by learning processes. We still do not believe that 'one off' test results can, in all cases, provide diagnostic criteria of a disease profile. This is particularly true of higher ability subjects who must 'pass through' the entire normal range before they show as statistically abnormal.

This work was undertaken by the Alzheimer Research Group of the Robens Institute at the University of Surrey (Robinson, personal communication).

CONCLUSIONS

Thus in conclusion, the dementias continue to present a tremendous challenge for the future to all those concerned with the most distressing of illnesses. A better understanding of measurement in the disease syndrome together with its natural histories, are essential if the newer promising drug therapies are to be evaluated in a timely and effective way.

REFERENCES

Alzheimer's Disease Society (1991). *Caring for the Person with Dementia—A Guide for Families and Other Carers.* Alzheimers Disease Society, London.

Arie, T. (1983). Dementia (review article). *Br. Med. J.,* **4**, 540–543.

Clarke, M., Jagger, C., Anderson, J., Battcock, T., Kelly, F. and Campbell Stern, M. (1991). The prevalence of dementia in a total population: a comparison of two screening instruments. *Age Aging,* **20**, 396–403.

Goodin, D.S. (1986). Event related endogenous potentials. In: Aminoff, M.J. (Ed.), *Electrodiagnosis in Clinical Neurology.* Churchill Livingstone, New York, pp. 575–595.

Goodin, D.S., Squires, K.C., Henderson, B.H. and Starr, A. (1978). Age related variations in evoked potentials to auditory stimuli in normal subjects. *Electroceph. Clin. Neurophysiol.,* **44**, 447–458.

Hachinski, V.C., Illife, L.D., Zilhka, E., Du Boulay, G.H., McAllister, V.L., Marshall, J., Ross Russell, R.W. and Symon, L. (1975). Cerebral blood flow in dementia. *Arch. Neurol.,* **32**, 632–636.

Mace, N.L., Rabins, P.V., Castleton, B., Cloke, C. and McEwen, E. (1990). *The 36-Hour Day. Caring at Home for Confused Elderly People.* Age Concern, London.

Moran, J. (1991). *Alzheimer's Disease: New Therapies and the World Market.* Management Report, Financial Times Business Information Ltd, London.

OCED (1987). *Financing and Delivering Healthcare: A Comparative Analysis of OCED Countries.* OCED, Paris.

Pfeffer, R.I., Afifi, A.A. and Chance, J.M. (1987). Prevalence of Alzheimer's disease in a retirement community. *Am. J. Epidemiol.,* **125**, 420–436.

Polich, J. (1987). Comparison of P300 from a passive tone sequence paradigm and an active discrimination task. *Psychophysiology,* **24**, 41–46.

Polich, J. (1989). P300 from a passive auditory paradigm. *Electroenceph. Clin. Neurophysiol.,* **74**, 312–320.

Sacks, O. (1991). *Alzheimer's Disease, Handbook for Carers.* Alzheimer's Society of Canada.

Squires, K.C., Chippendale, T.J., Wrege, K.W., Goodin, D.S. and Starr, A. (1980). Electrophysiological assessment of mental function in aging and dementia. In: Poon, L. (Ed.), *Aging in the 1980s.* American Psychological Association, Washington, DC, pp. 125–134.

Sutton, S., Braren, M., Zubin, J. and John, E.R. (1965). Evoked potential correlates of stimulus uncertainty. *Science*, **150**, 1187–1188.

WHO Regional Office for Europe (1989) *Monitoring of the Strategy for Health for All by the Year 2000. Part 1: The Situation in the European Region, 1987/88.* WHO, Copenhagen.

The Management of Alzheimer's Disease
Edited by Gordon K. Wilcock
©1993 Wrightson Biomedical Publishing Ltd

4

Imaging in Alzheimer's Disease

DAVID KATZ

*Consultant Radiologist, Northwick Park Hospital and Clinical Research Centre,
Harrow, UK*

INTRODUCTION

Imaging techniques are likely to play an increasing role in the diagnosis and assessment of patients with Alzheimer's disease (AD). Histological diagnosis made at autopsy is the 'gold standard' for confirming the disease, but as technology advances it seems reasonable to expect that imaging will develop and allow a similar degree of diagnostic accuracy (Albert and Lafleche, 1991).

Imaging not only allows diagnosis and monitoring of the progression of AD but may reveal focal disorders and other potentially treatable causes of dementia.

The following discussion describes the technology used at present and the relative merits of each modality.

Imaging techniques provide both structural and functional information about the brain.

Computed tomography (CT) and magnetic resonance imaging (MRI) display structured detail of the brain and will often reveal causes of dementia such as cerebral infarction, tumour, subdural haematomas and hydrocephalus.

Functional techniques such as single photon emission computed tomography (SPECT) and positron emission tomography (PET) provide physiological data and will reveal for example information on regional blood flow and cerebral metabolic rates for glucose and oxygen.

COMPUTED TOMOGRAPHY

Computed tomography (CT) produces cross-sectional images of the brain. A narrow beam of X-rays is emitted from an X-ray tube which rotates around

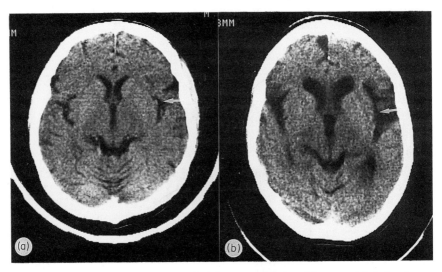

Figure 1. (a) Normal CT appearance in 71 year old male with normal Sylvian fissure (arrow). (b) 60 year old male with Alzheimer's disease illustrating global atrophy with ventricular enlargement. Grossly dilated Sylvian fissure (arrow) indicates marked temporal lobe atrophy.

the head. The X-rays are transmitted through the brain and differentially absorbed. The emerging attenuated beam is measured by detectors and computers then recreate an axial image of brain structures.

AD produces cell loss and brain shrinkage. Although the plaques and tangles that are the histological hallmark of the disease (Khatchaturian, 1985) cannot be seen on CT, atrophic change that is a reflection of the destruction of brain tissue can be measured (Fig. 1).

Cortical atrophy and ventricular enlargement are prominent features of AD. It is important to bear in mind (1) that early in AD there may be little or no atrophy and (2) that atrophy also may occur in dementia of other causes as well as in normal ageing patients (Fazekas *et al.*, 1987). The rate of enlargement of the lateral ventricles is a sensitive measure used to differentiate AD from controls (Luxenberg *et al.*, 1987).

Global atrophy and ventricular enlargement are not specific markers in AD but there is evidence that suggests that regional atrophy particularly in the temporal lobes may distinguish AD from other atrophic causes (Kido *et al.*, 1989).

CT is often used in differential diagnosis to determine whether other structural causes for dementia are present. Mass lesions and large infarcts are readily distinguished but small (lacunar) infarcts that are associated with multi-infarct dementia (MID) are often difficult to define due to the limited degree of contrast sensitivity (Johnson *et al.*, 1987).

CT is widely available, is relatively inexpensive and as an adjunct to clinical assessment has become a mainstay of diagnosis of the dementia syndromes.

MAGNETIC RESONANCE IMAGING

Magnetic resonance imaging (MRI) uses magnetic fields to obtain images of body structures. MRI technology is based on the fact that atoms whose nuclei have an odd number of protons or neutrons have an electrical charge and act as magnets. The atoms, which are normally randomly arranged, align themselves uniformly when a strong magnetic field is applied across them. If a radiowave is then aimed at an angle to the magnetic field the nuclei flip out of alignment. When the radiowave is switched off the nuclei 'relax' and realign themselves with the magnetic field and emit an electromagnetic wave of the same frequency as the radiowave. The computer measures the electromagnetic waves and constructs a composite picture.

As water is the most common molecule in the body, the MRI signal effectively measures the electromagnetic waves emitted by the hydrogen atoms in water. Because grey matter, white matter and CSF contain varying amounts of water the MRI computer can distinguish them from each other and construct a detailed image of the brain.

MRI has much better contrast sensitivity and spatial resolution than CT. MRI also allows visualization of the brain in multiple planes and has the added advantage of not using ionizing radiation.

White matter hyperintensities seen in the subcortical white matter and in the periventricular region may reflect infarction or other tissue changes that may be present in vascular dementia, AD or normal ageing (Jernigan *et al.*, 1990). White matter lesions are present in all patients with multi-infarct dementia (MID) but their presence does not preclude the diagnosis of AD (Erkinjuntti *et al.*, 1984) (see Figs 2–4).

The high contrast resolution available with MRI enables accurate identification of brain structures. Studies comparing the size of the hippocampus in AD with age matched controls suggests that AD can be identified without overlap and this may well become a useful diagnostic tool (Seab *et al.*, 1988). General atrophy seen on MRI has the same problems and is no more useful than the atrophy seen on CT.

MRI is more sensitive than CT in revealing structural lesions but, at present, the advantages gained from this in diagnosing AD are still somewhat equivocal. MRI remains relatively expensive and is much less widely available than CT.

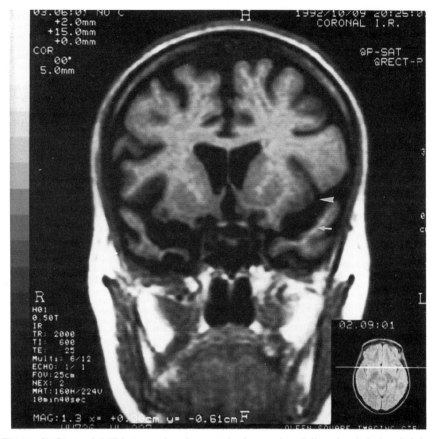

Figure 2. Coronal MRI scan showing marked atrophy. Dilatation of the Sylvian fissure (arrow head) with grossly atrophic hippocampus (arrow).

Further research will no doubt improve our understanding of the significance of the many changes seen on MRI.

FUNCTIONAL (NUCLEAR) IMAGING

Radionuclide imaging is based on the ability to detect electromagnetic radiation emitted from an injected radioactive tracer that has been taken up by the organ to be studied. The radiation emitted is absorbed by a detector. The information from the detector is digitized and fed to a computer that eventually produces an image which can be interpreted by the clinicians.

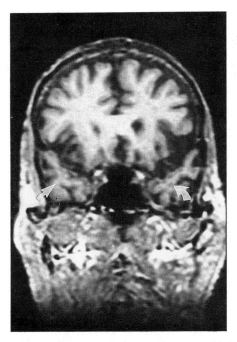

Figure 3. Coronal MRI scan showing symmetrical temporal lobe atrophy which may be seen in Alzheimer's disease. The atrophy on the left side (curved arrow) is much more marked than on the right (straight arrow).

Imaging the isotope distribution in a single plane is useful but there can be difficulty in interpreting images due to overlapping activity from superimposed tissues. To overcome this problem, sectional images can be obtained by emission computed tomography (ECT). Information is gathered from all around the patient and the computer reconstructs the images that represent slices through the patient. ECT yields images without overlapping counts from the radioactivity in adjacent areas or background tissues. This attribute increases contrast tissue resolution (i.e. the ability to discern differences in tracer concentration in neighbouring tissue) (Costa and Ell, 1991).

There are two types of ECT in use: (1) single photon emission computed tomography (SPECT) and (2) positron emission tomography (PET). Both techniques are similar in the images they produce and in the methods of reconstruction but they differ in the method used to collect photons. Detection counters are mounted on a gantry. The counters may be fixed or may rotate around the imaging table over an arc of at least 180°. The computer is used to reconstruct images that represent slices through the patient perpendicular to the axis of rotation.

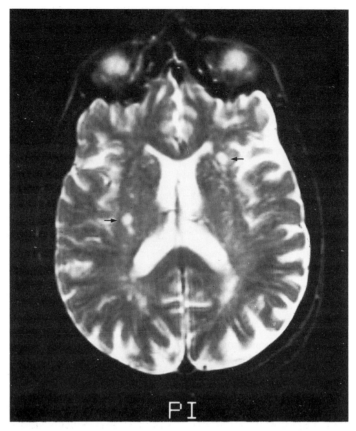

Figure 4. Axial MRI scan showing several high signal lesions (arrows) indicating small infarcts. These lesions were not seen on CT scan and suggest multi-infarct dementia.

Positron emission tomography

PET images use high energy photons that are emitted at an 180° angle to each other upon annihilation of a positron. This allows simultaneous detection of the two photons in opposing detectors which provides high detection efficiency and good uniform resolution.

Radionuclides used in PET are cyclotron produced. They are unstable and have short half lives and therefore must be produced by a cyclotron on site. The cost of purchasing and maintaining a dedicated cyclotron is prohibitive in most clinical settings.

The radionuclide which has been most commonly used in PET and AD is ^{18}F-fluorodeoxyglucose which measures glucose metabolism. Increases in brain activity produce increases in glucose metabolism. There is a differential decline in glucose metabolism in the association cortices in patients with AD and the greatest decline is in the inferior parietal cortex and temporal cortex. The decline seen in mildly impaired patients is much less striking than in more severely affected patients (Chase *et al.*, 1984).

Studies comparing AD with MID show that AD patients have large regional declines whereas MID patients have scattered focal defects. However, as with the structural imaging techniques there tends to be overlap among the dementias. For example parietal hypometabolism is typical of AD but may also be seen in Parkinsons disease (Jagust *et al.*, 1990).

Single photon emission computer tomography

The radionuclides used in SPECT are single photon or gamma emitters as opposed to the positron emitters used in PET. In SPECT the tracer used must label a compound that is recognized by metabolic or enzymatic receptor sites—a process that may be inefficient and difficult. SPECT's advantages over PET are that the radioactive markers are more stable and can be sold commercially and are much less expensive. The disadvantage of SPECT in relation to PET is its lower spatial resolution (Albert *et al.*, 1990).

The radioactive tracers that have been used primarily in AD are *n*-isopropyl *n*-iodoamphetamine (IMP) labelled with ^{123}I and hexamethyl propyleneamine oxime (HMPAO) labelled with ^{99m}Tc. Both are distributed in proportion to cerebral blood flow. Like PET, SPECT reveals reductions in blood flow predominantly in the temporo-parietal region. The front cover of this book shows axial (left) and coronal (right) SPECT scans demonstrating reduced blood flow (arrows) in the temporal lobes. Decrease in cerebral blood flow in these areas is usually symmetrical although asymmetrical patterns have also been reported. The current data indicate that moderately and severely impaired patients with AD can be differentiated from controls with a relatively high degree of accuracy with SPECT. Studies of mildly impaired patients are associated with a much lower degree of accuracy (Johnson *et al.*, 1988; Reed *et al.*, 1989).

CONCLUSION

Both the structural and functional imaging techniques discussed differentiate severely to moderately impaired patients with substantial accuracy but negative imaging does not rule out the diagnosis of AD.

At present it seems prudent to exclude a treatable cause of dementia syndromes with an anatomical imaging technique.

All of the modalities described have limitations however and the diagnosis of AD remains a clinical diagnosis and none of the techniques can supplant careful clinical examination of the demented patient.

REFERENCES

Albert, M.S. and Lafleche, G. (1991). Neuroimaging in Alzheimer's disease. *Psychiatr. Clinics N. Am.*, **14**, 443–459.

Albert, M.S., Duffy, F.H. and McAnulty, G.B. (1990). Electrophysiologic comparisons between two groups of patients with Alzheimer's disease. *Arch. Neurol*, **47**, 857–863.

Chase, T.N., Foster, N.C.L., Fedio, P., Brooks, R., Mansi, L. and Chiro, G.D. (1984). Regional cortical dysfunction in Alzheimer's disease as determined by positron emission tomography. *Ann. Neurol*, **15** (Suppl. 1), 5170–5174.

Costa, D.C. and Ell, P.J. (1991). *Brain Blood Flow in Neurology & Psychiatry*. Churchill Livingstone, New York.

Erkinjuntti, T., Sipponen, J.T., Iivanainen, M., Ketonen, L., Sulkava, R. and Sepponen, R.E. (1984). Cerebral NMR and CT imaging in dementia. *J. Comput. Assist. Tomogr.*, **8**, 614–618.

Fazekas, F., Chawluk, J.B., Alavi, A., Hurtig, H.I. and Zimmerman, R.A. (1987). MR signal abnormalities at 1.5T in Alzheimer's dementia and normal aging. *Am. J. Neuroradiol.*, **8**, 421–426.

Jagust, W.J., Reed, B.R., Seab, J.P. and Bodinger, T.F. (1990). Alzheimer's disease: age at onset and single-photon emission computed tomographic patterns of regional cerebral blood flow. *Arch. Neurol*, **47**, 628–633.

Jernigan, T.L., Press, G.A. and Hesselink, J.R. (1990). Methods for measuring brain morphologic features on magnetic resonance images. *Arch. Neurol.*, **47**, 27–32.

Johnson, K.A., Davis, K.R., Buonanno, F.S., Brady, T.J., Rosen, J. and Growdon, J.H. (1987). Comparison of magnetic resonance and roentgen ray computed tomography in dementia. *Arch. Neurol*, **44**, 1075–1080.

Johnson, K.A., Holman, B.L., Mueller, S.P., Rosen, T.J., English, R., Nagel, J.S. and Growdon, J.H. (1988). Single photon emission computed tomography in Alzheimer's disease. *Arch. Neurol.*, **45**, 392–396.

Khatchaturian, Z. (1985). Diagnosis of Alzheimer's disease. *Arch. Neurol.*, **42**, 1097–1105.

Kido, D.K., Caine, E.D., Lemay, M., Ekholm, S., Booth, H. and Panzer, R. (1989). Temporal lobe atrophy in patients with Alzheimer's disease. *Am. J. Neuroradiol.*, **10**, 551–556.

Luxenberg, J.S., Haxby, J.V., Creasey, H., Sundaram, M. and Raporort, S.I. (1987). Rate of ventricular enlargement in dementia of the Alzheimer type correlates with rate of neuropsychological deterioration. *Neurology*, **37**, 1135–1140.

Reed, P.R., Jagust, W.J., Seab, J.P. and Ober, B.A. (1989). Memory and regional cerebral blood flow in mildly symptomatic Alzheimer's disease. *Neurology*, **39**, 1537–1539.

Seab, J.P., Jagust, W.J., Wong, S.T.S., Roos, M.S., Reed, B.R. and Budinger, T.F. (1988). Quantitative NMR measurements of hippocampal atrophy in Alzheimer's disease. *Magn. Reson. Med.*, **8**, 200–208.

5

What Can be Treated in Alzheimer's Disease?

ROGER BRIGGS

Professor of Geriatric Medicine, University of Southampton, UK

INTRODUCTION

'What can be treated in Alzheimer's disease?' At first sight, this seems a straightforward 'medical question', and the truthful answer given the current state of knowledge might be 'not much'. The search for effective treatments in Alzheimer's disease (AD) is still guided by observations, made some 15 years ago, of defects in the central cholinergic system. However, other neurotransmitter systems are also affected in AD, and the clinical features are not confined to impairments of learning and memory (Briggs, 1989).

Current research is tending to concentrate on the basic mechanisms underlying the development of the pathology of AD, at molecular and cellular level and in terms of neuronal organization within the brain. Obviously, it is to be hoped that the 'cause' of AD can be found and preventative strategies developed: several of the chapters in this book address the problem of AD from the 'medical model' standpoint. The traditional distinction between 'ageing' and 'disease' may well be inappropriate, particularly when applied to 'senile dementia' (Grimley Evans, 1990), but it is worth recalling some aspects of the epidemiology of dementia. It is well known that the prevalence of AD increases with age, though it is less certain whether incidence rises in similar fashion. If incidence does continue to increase with age, Jorm (1990) has demonstrated that the overall lifetime risk of the development of AD would approach 100% (see also Chapter 1). Could cognitive decline be an inevitable feature of the human condition, given a long enough lifespan?

For the time being, we are faced with the challenge of looking after the many sufferers from AD and their carers. The 'social' aspects of the management of dementia are also the topic of several contributions to this book. In this chapter, I will illustrate the complementary nature of different theoretical perspectives by drawing on biological, psychological and sociological approaches to the treatment of Alzheimer's disease.

LOSS OF SELF

During the search for drug treatments of dementia, psychologists have played a major role in the development of tools for the ascertainment of dementia and the assessment of its severity. More recently, psychological interest has broadened to encompass some understanding of what it may mean to an individual to experience a dementing process, and to explore possibilities of therapeutic intervention. To concentrate merely on cognitive failure is inadequate: what is it like to listen to a close relative whom one has loved for years, but no longer to understand what they are saying or possibly even to recognize who they are? It is hard for those of us who try to help dementing people to appreciate how devastating such 'loss of self' must be (Gilleard, 1984).

Observations of people in the early stage of dementia reveal considerable self-awareness and insight (Froggatt, 1988). Although much research and practical effort is concentrated on carers in need of support, relatively little importance is attached to the subjective experience of dementing people themselves. Might not a better understanding of that experience help to retain a sense of self, by 'maintaining emotional health around the cognitive impairment'? It is important to reinforce the remaining abilities of a dementing subject, not just to focus on their disabilities. Approaches such as reality orientation (Holden and Woods, 1988) and reminiscence (Coleman, 1986) are examples of 'therapies' which attempt to maintain cognitively impaired people in contact with ordinary daily events, and their past lives. It is difficult to demonstrate that treatments of this type are 'effective' in a conventional medical sense, since such individualized interventions are not easily fitted into the framework of the double-blind, placebo-controlled trial. Experimental designs suitable for single case studies may be more appropriate (Garland, 1990).

A lifespan perspective can help us to understand an individual's behaviours and the cues to which he or she responds in terms of habits developed through earlier experience. It has even been argued that social and psychological factors may play a part in the aetiology of dementia (Kitwood, 1988). According to this view, dementia might be understood, psychologically, as the consequence of the removal of the main cognitive supports that had preserved a person's sense of self: neuropathological consequences could arise from social and psychological roots such as loss of roles, impoverishment of social life, and so on. 'Dementia is an existential plight of persons—not simply a problem to be investigated and managed through technical skill.'

Those of us who work at the biomedical end of the spectrum may find it hard to come to terms with the extremity of the underlying hypothesis but few, surely, can carp at the sentiment of the quoted conclusion. We are well used to taking cognisance of psychosocial factors in the genesis and treatment of heart disease and cancer, so why not for diseases which affect the brain and mind directly?

DEPRESSION AND DEMENTIA

Subtle cognitive impairment (or the subjective complaint of memory problems) may be a feature of depressive illness in old age. Much emphasis has been placed on the diagnostic difficulties theoretically posed by elderly depressed patients in whom prominent cognitive dysfunction is the essential clinical feature, those with 'depressive pseudodementia'. Kral and Emery (1989) followed up 44 such patients (mean age 76.5 years) for an average of eight years: although all subjects responded well to antidepressant treatment initially, 89% subsequently developed clinical dementia of the Alzheimer type.

Depression may not only mimic or presage AD, but may also complicate the disease early or late in its course (Katona, 1991). In a review of several studies (Wragg and Jeste, 1989), depressed mood was recorded in 0–87% (median 41%) and depressive disorder in 0–86% (median 19%) of patients with established AD. In most studies, depressed mood was commoner in the Alzheimer's subjects than in healthy elderly controls. The excess prevalence of depressive symptoms in AD is not surprising whether one attributes their development to loss of biogenic amines, life events or both.

Greenwald and colleagues (1989) studied a group of dementing patients with coexistent depression (dementia/depression) compared with elderly inpatients with a major depressive episode only (depression-only) or dementia-only. Dementia/depression patients were distinguished from the other two groups by greater feelings of self-pity and sensitivity to rejection, but shared many classical depressive features with the depression-only group (not manifest in the dementia-only group). Persistent and aggressive treatment with sequential trials of antidepressants (including tricyclics), and electroconvulsive therapy (ECT) in some patients, showed a similar response of depressive symptoms in the dementia/depression group (70% responded) and the depression-only group (73% responded). In the patients with coexistent syndromes, depression appeared to interact with dementia to lower performance on cognitive tests. Although remaining in the severely impaired range, this performance improved in the dementia/depression group following antidepressant treatment; no cognitive improvement was seen in the dementia-only group, arguing against non-specific environmental or psychological effects of the hospital regime.

The above study was prospective, but included relatively small numbers of patients, with diagnoses of either probable AD or multi-infarct dementia; treatment regimes were not standardized. Nevertheless, the findings are in line with several anecdotal reports describing concomitant improvements in mood and cognition following antidepressant therapy in demented patients with superimposed depression. This is despite the facts that tricyclic drugs might be expected to exacerbate any 'cholinergic deficit' in Alzheimer's disease, and that ECT may induce acute impairments of memory. The pharmacological treatment of depression in dementia is surely an area where standardized, double-blind, placebo-controlled trials could usefully be applied.

For a further discussion of depression, the reader is referred to Chapter 8.

ACUTE CONFUSIONAL STATES

The term 'acute confusional state' (or 'delirium') implies a temporary disturbance of intellectual function, usually of rapid onset over hours or days. An episode of acute confusion is represented schematically in Fig. 1. The key points to note are the abrupt decline in someone whose mental function was previously good, and the return of cognitive function after the episode is over (Briggs, 1985).

Such episodes are characterized by clouded consciousness, disorientation, illusions and often vivid hallucinations; fluctuating state of awareness is accompanied by sleep–wake disruption and nocturnal worsening of

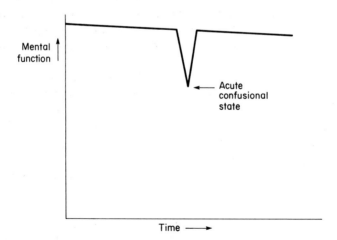

Figure 1. Schematic representation of acute confusional state.

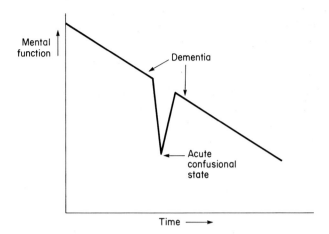

Figure 2. Acute confusional state superimposed on a dementing process.

symptoms. Lipowski (1988) suggests that the term 'delirium' should be restricted to transient cognitive disorders of organic aetiology, to the exclusion of similar symptoms of functional origin. Acute confusional states are usually due to some toxic or metabolic process, illness affecting the brain or other organs, and are often reversible. By analogy with other systems (cardiac and renal, for example) some clinicians call delirium 'acute brain failure'.

Ageing may itself increase susceptibility to acute confusional states (Burrows *et al.*, 1985), not merely because the elderly are more liable to suffer from serious physical illness. However, subjects with structural brain diseases (including AD) have a marked predisposition to the development of delirium (Kopenen *et al.*, 1989). Figure 2 represents an episode of acute confusion occurring in the context of a dementing process ('acute on chronic brain failure').

It is important to realize that a sudden change in behaviour of a dementing person is likely to be a non-specific presentation of a physical illness. An acute confusional state may make it quite impossible to support such a person at home; appropriate diagnosis and treatment may enable them to be cared for in the community again.

Virtually any illness, and many drugs, may induce delirium in a dementing elderly subject: some examples are shown in Table 1, but the list is by no means comprehensive.

Urinary tract infection and pneumonia are common precipitants of an acute confusional state, often without specific symptoms or marked pyrexia. Simple diagnostic aids (such as testing for proteinuria or measuring respiratory rate) may give helpful clues. Congestive cardiac failure is also a frequent

Table 1. Causes of acute confusional state with examples
shown in parentheses

Infective	(respiratory or urinary tract infection)
Cardiac	(heart failure, myocardial infarction)
Metabolic	(electrolyte disturbance)
Neurological	(stroke, post-ictal state)
Endocrine	(diabetes, thyroid disease)
Nutritional	(cachexia, thiamine deficiency)
Drugs	(antidepressants, anticonvulsants, sedatives)
Miscellaneous	(trauma, sudden isolation)

cause of delirium—but so is over-vigorous use of diuretics leading to electrolyte disturbance. Myocardiac infarction may present without typical cardiac pain, the evidence only coming to light on an electrocardiograph. Diabetes and thyroid disease are both more prevalent in the elderly than in the young, and are often screened for in dementia. However, they may coexist with AD, so that treatment of the endocrine disorder does not always lead to any improvement in cognitive function. Although senile dementia predisposes to malnutrition, it is unusual for specific dietary deficiencies (of thiamine, for example) to be of clinical significance in AD. Patients with Alzheimer's disease do tend to lose weight, particularly later in the course of the disease, for reasons which are not certain (Prentice *et al.*, 1989). The benefits of nutritional intervention are not established. Those who suffer from AD are not immune to cancer, and the possibility of an underlying malignancy should be borne in mind if weight loss and deterioration in general health seem out of proportion to the degree of dementia.

Almost all drugs that are prescribed for their actions on the central nervous system (such as sedatives, tranquillizers, antidepressants, anticonvulsants, anti-Parkinsonian agents) and many others (such as some antibiotics, digoxin) may cause confusion as a side-effect. Once a patient has developed delirium, it is often best to withdraw all drugs to see if the patient improves. It is rare that withdrawal of medication leads to immediate problems (though caution is needed with some drugs such as steroids). If diuretics are stopped, for example, they can always be reinstituted if signs of heart failure appear.

Some geriatricians believe that constipation may cause confusion in dementing subjects; whether this is true or not, faecal impaction can certainly add to distress and discomfort, and may well lead to faecal incontinence. Accidental trauma, surgery and general anaesthesia, singly or in concert, may precipitate delirium which persists for several days; falls (and hip fractures) are common in AD. Emotional trauma (sudden isolation, a bereavement, or a burglary) may further unbalance a mind already on the verge of collapse.

The admission to hospital of a confused elderly patient will, of course, increase the bewilderment and disorientation which they already suffer.

From the above it follows that a clinical examination and some basic investigations (urinalysis, blood tests, electrocardiogram and chest X-ray) will often reveal the cause of an acute confusional state. It should be noted that investigations directed specifically at the central nervous system are not usually indicated (unless mandated by focal neurological signs, meningism or the like). In real life, the situation is often not clear-cut—one is faced with an old lady brought into casualty after a fall, who cannot give a history, has six bottles of pills in her handbag, crepitations at both lung bases, sugar in her urine, and a fractured neck of femur. The practical solution is to treat the obvious and hope for the best.

Finally, I have dealt with 'delirium' and 'dementia' as if they are two clinically distinct syndromes, but which may occur together. Whilst it is convenient for operational reasons to think in these terms ('dementia' requires long-term management; 'delirium' is a medical emergency), there is in fact a considerable degree of overlap, as has been pointed out by Pitt (1991).

CARER'S PROBLEMS

The mainstay of the management of dementia in the community is support for caring relatives. This requires adequate provision of community psychiatric nurses, day hospitals and centres, social services and relative support groups; all of these must be coordinated effectively. The aim must be to sustain the morale and the capacity to cope of the carers, responding flexibly to their needs before crises develop. Intermittent respite care may provide a much-needed break. However, community care is not always sufficient, particularly when the carer has had a poor relationship with the sufferer even before the onset of dementia. Many old people have no close relatives to support them and it may be difficult (and sometimes inhumane) to leave them to a precarious existence alone at home; dementia is thus the principal reason for admission to long-term institutional care. A number of authors in this book go into these aspects of the management of dementia in some detail (see Chapters 11 and 12). For the remainder of this chapter, I will allude to those problems most commonly faced by carers.

A study by Argyle and colleagues (1985) reviewed patients who had been admitted to a psychogeriatric unit because their relatives could no longer cope at home, to determine the number and nature of problems and how well these problems were tolerated. The average number of problems reported by carers was high (12.3) with behavioural problems being the most prominent. Table 2 shows the difficulties most frequently experienced by carers, but which they claimed to cope with well.

Table 2. Carer's problems—well tolerated.

	Percentage of carers reporting problem
Reduced social life	74%
Embarrassment	58%
Anxiety or depression	51%
Dressing	69%
Washing	48%
Urinary incontinence	50%

(After Argyle *et al.*, 1985.)

Most carers have to put up with a reduced social life and some embarrassment, but do so with good grace. A number of carers develop psychological symptoms of anxiety or depression themselves. Accurate and timely information concerning the nature of dementia and the support services which are available enable carers to deal with their situation much better; knowing about a service such as respite care may help them to carry on even if the service is not used. As well as support and counselling, a minority of carers may need treatment with psychotropic drugs.

Practical solutions, such as providing a laundry service, may seem obvious for some problems but efficient provision of help depends upon proper assessment of need. For example, difficulty with dressing is common in AD, but can reflect a number of underlying disabilities—not being able to remember what to wear, not being able to work out the right movement in order to put the clothing on, or straightforward physical limitations. An occupational therapist may well be able to teach the carer strategies to overcome such difficulties, even if the dementing person is unable to learn.

Urinary incontinence commonly develops during the course of AD. Remediable causes such as urinary tract infection, faecal impaction, stress incontinence or prostatic disease should be sought and treated, but in many cases urge incontinence is due to failure of neurological control resulting in bladder detrusor instability. A variety of treatment approaches are available, some more likely to succeed than others in the context of an underlying dementia (Ouslander, 1990). Behaviourally oriented procedures which are dependent on the patient, including biofeedback and bladder retraining, require adequate cognitive function and motivation. Habit training relies on the care-giver to institute and reinforce a suitably structured toileting regime. The goal of preventing wetting episodes can sometimes be achieved, but the process can also lead to friction between sufferer and carer. A fixed toileting schedule may work better in these circumstances, the clock rather than the carer taking the blame for what can seem like nagging. Imipramine or other anticholinergic drugs may also be useful adjuncts, side-effects permitting.

Table 3. Carer's problems—poorly tolerated.

	Percentage of carers reporting problem
Aggression	35%
Verbal abuse	27%
Wandering	30%
Faecal smearing	23%
Inappropriate urination	24%
Sleep disturbance	48%
Restless by day	52%

(After Argyle *et al.*, 1985.)

However, even a combined behavioural and pharmacological approach to the treatment of urge incontinence is less likely to be effective the more severe is the patient's cognitive impairment (Castleden *et al.*, 1985).

The common problems with which carers find it difficult or impossible to cope are shown in Table 3: 'physical aggression, verbal abuse, wandering, inappropriate urination and faecal smearing, the problems that nobody likes to talk about' (Argyle *et al.*, 1985). These are behavioural problems which are very difficult to modify but which put an enormous burden on the carer and occasionally lead to verbal or physical abuse of the dementing person. Provision of adequate support facilities is, of course, the best method of preventing abuse (Bennett, 1990). Psychotropic drugs including phenothiazines and depot neuroleptics are frequently used to control agitation, restlessness and aggression, but dosage must be carefully monitored to avoid excessive sedation or further impairment of cognitive functionand mobility. Thioridazine is widely used though there is no substantial evidence that it is superior to other similar agents.

Choice of a suitable hypnotic may also be difficult, but carers need to get adequate sleep themselves if they are to cope. Drugs with a relatively short half-life (such as temazepam or chlormethiazole) are often prescribed, though no drug will be appropriate to all cases.

Although restlessness and wandering give rise to problems earlier in the course of AD, by the late stages falls and immobility may be prominent. The role of physiotherapy in the management of elderly people with dementia has been little evaluated so far, and appropriate measures of mobility skills are only now being developed (Pomeroy, 1990).

CONCLUSION

'What can be treated in Alzheimer's disease?' It is greatly to be hoped that research will lead to drugs effective against the core symptoms of AD, which can halt progression of the pathological process or even prevent it altogether. Meanwhile, sufferers and their carers require the integrated provision of a diagnostic service, community support and institutional care of a high standard. General practitioners have a key role in orchestrating a comprehensive medical and social response to a dementing patient (Philp, 1989). I have taken a broad view of what constitutes 'treatment': even when doctors can prescribe effective drugs, there is a place for a range of psychological, behavioural, and environmental interventions to address the problems of people who suffer and those who care for them. This is reflected in the breadth of topics covered in this book, and in the diverse backgrounds of the authors. Both research into Alzheimer's disease and its management are complex, benefitting from the cooperation of many disciplines. Alzheimer's disease is a model of what makes care of the elderly such a challenging and rewarding endeavour.

REFERENCES

Argyle, N., Jestice, S. and Brook, C.P.B. (1985). Psychogeriatric patients: their supporters' problems. *Age Ageing*, **14**, 355–360.

Bennett, G.C. (1990). Abuse of the elderly: prevention and legislation. *Geriatr. Med.*, **20**, 55–60.

Briggs, R. (1985). Acute confusion. In: Lye, M. (Ed.), *Acute Geriatric Medicine*. MTP Press, Lancaster, pp. 113–134.

Briggs, R.S.J. (1989). Alzheimer's disease: the clinical context. In: Davies, D.C. (Ed.), *Alzheimer's Disease: Towards an Understanding of the Aetiology and Pathogenesis*. John Libbey, London, pp. 1–7.

Burrows, J., Briggs, R.S. and Elkington, A.R. (1985). Cataract extraction and confusion in elderly patients. *J. Clin. Exp. Gerontol.*, **7**, 51–70.

Castleden, C.M., Duffin, H.M., Asher, M.J. and Yeomanson, C.W. (1985). Factors influencing outcome in elderly patient with urinary incontinence and detrusor instability. *Age Ageing*, **14**, 303–307.

Coleman, P.G. (1986). *Ageing and Reminiscence Processes: Social and Clinical Implications*. Wiley, Chichester.

Froggatt, A. (1988). Self-awareness in early dementia. In: Gearing, B., Johnson, M. and Heller, T. (Eds), *Mental Health Problems in Old Age*, Wiley, Chichester, pp. 131–136.

Garland, J.G. (1990). Environment and behaviour: a clinical perspective. In: Bond, J. and Coleman, P. (Eds), *Ageing in Society: An Introduction to Social Gerontology*. Sage, London, pp. 123–143.

Gilleard, C.J. (1984). *Living with Dementia: Community Care of the Elderly Mentally Infirm*. Croom Helm, London.

Greenwald, B.S., Kramer-Ginsberg, E., Marin, D.B., Laitman, L.B., Hermann, C.K., Mohs, R.C. and Davis, K.L. (1989). Dementia with coexistent major depression. *Am. J. Psychiatry*, **146**, 1472–1478.

Grimley Evans, J. (1990). How are the elderly different? In: Kane, R.L., Evans, J.G. and MacFadyen, D. (Eds), *Improving the Health of Older People: A World View*. Oxford University Press, Oxford, pp. 50–68.

Holden, U.P. and Woods, R.T. (1988). *Reality Orientation: Psychological Approaches to the Confused Elderly.* Churchill Livingstone, Edinburgh.

Jorm, A.F. (1990). *The Epidemiology of Alzheimer's Disease and Related Disorders.* Chapman and Hall, London.

Katona, C.L.E. (1991). Depression in old age. *Rev. Clin. Gerontol.*, **1**, 371–384.

Kitwood, T. (1988). The contribution of psychology to the understanding of senile dementia. In: Gearing, B., Johnson, M. and Heller, T. (Eds), *Mental Health Problems in Old Age*, Wiley, Chichester, pp. 123–130.

Kopenen, H., Hurri, L., Stenback, U., Mattila, E., Soininen, H. and Reikkinen, P.J. (1989). Computed tomography findings in delirium. *J. Nerv. Ment. Dis.*, **177**, 226–231.

Kral, V.A. and Emery, O.B. (1989). Long-term follow-up of depressive pseudodementia of the aged. *Can. J. Psychiatry*, **34**, 445–446.

Lipowski, Z.J. (1988). Transient cognitive disorders (delirium, acute confusional states) in the elderly. *Am. J. Psychiatry*, **140**, 1426–1436.

Ouslander, J.G. (1990). The efficacy of continence treatment. In: Kane, R.L., Evans, J.G. and MacFadyen, D. (Eds), *Improving the Health of Older People: A World View.* Oxford University Press, Oxford, pp. 273–295.

Philp, I. (1989). Challenge of dementia to the GP: five areas of attack. *Geriatr. Med.*, **19**, 19–25.

Pitt, B. (1991). Delirium. *Rev. Clin. Gerontol.*, **1**, 147–157.

Pomeroy, V. (1990). Development of an ADL oriented assessment-of-mobility scale suitable for use with elderly people with dementia. *Physiotherapy*, **76**, 446–448.

Prentice, A.M., Leavesley, K., Murgatroyd, P.R., Coward, W.A., Schorah, C.J., Bladon, P.T. and Hullin, R.P. (1989). Is severe wasting in elderly mental patients caused by an excessive energy requirement? *Age Ageing*, **18**, 158–167.

Wragg, R.E. and Jeste, D.V. (1989). Overview of depression and psychosis in Alzheimer's disease. *Am. J. Psychiatry*, **136**, 577–587.

III
Management

The Management of Alzheimer's Disease
Edited by Gordon K. Wilcock
©1993 Wrightson Biomedical Publishing Ltd

6

The Role of the General Practitioner and Other Professionals in the Management of Alzheimer's Disease

MARGARET BLOOM

General Practitioner, London, UK

INTRODUCTION

Care for the chronically sick within the community has been the stated policy of successive governments in the UK for many years. As the elderly with dementia are particularly sensitive to their environment this seems to be in line with the best interests of the patients themselves.

However, the needs of the dementia patient are numerous and unless multiple services are available in adequate quantity, the lot of the patient and his family can be a miserable one. When faced with the tragedy of dementia the general practitioner (GP) will need to muster a variety of skills—the traditional ones of the personal and family physician, together with the modern ones of resource management and the ability to work effectively in a team.

IDENTIFYING THE CHALLENGE

The first task is to define the size of the problem within a particular practice. To this end prevalence data (i.e. the number of people who have a given condition at any one time) are of practical value. Estimates for the prevalence of dementia in the UK have varied considerably between studies. Although all agree that there is an increasing incidence with increasing age, it is now considered that some past estimates may have been too high (Copeland, 1990). Ineichen (1987) reviewed studies of prevalence in people over 65 years taking a restricted definition of dementia, which was thought

Table 1. Ineichen's rule-of-thumb for the
prevalence of dementia.

Age (years)	Prevalence (%)
65–74	1
75 and over	10

Reproduced with permission, from Ineichen (1987).

to be the most useful. He concluded that 2.8–2.9% of that population has moderate or severe dementia. His rule of thumb gives a simple and clear picture of the prevalence under and over 75 years (Table 1). A more recent study by O'Connor *et al.* (1989) broadly confirms these data. If early dementia is included, the figure is higher.

Thus a GP knowing his list size and age distribution can simply calculate the scale of the potential problem within his practice. He can then audit his

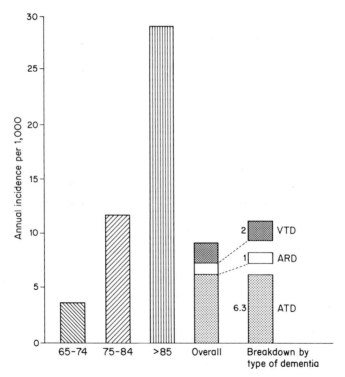

Figure 1. Incidence of dementia in the elderly and very elderly and the overall breakdown by type of dementia. (ATD, Alzheimer's type dementia; ARD, alcohol related dementia; VTD, vascular type dementia.) Reproduced with permission, from Laing and Hall (1991).

degree of success at identifying the group in need and plan how best to provide care. It is possible that one partner may have an interest in chronic illness or mental disease, but if not it is essential that an individual GP takes overall responsibility and has the main contact with a particular patient and that other partners, practice receptionists, and both formal and informal carers are aware of who this is. A working relationship of commitment and support must be entered into and haphazard arrangements involving many different GPs has no place in this often delicately balanced situation. Three main types of dementia are recognized, i.e. alcohol related, vascular due to multiple infarct or arterial disease, and Alzheimer's disease (Fig. 1), although some authorities now claim that the second commonest form of dementia is that caused by Lewy bodies.

It can be seen from Fig. 1 that Alzheimer's disease is the major cause of dementia in the elderly. From the perspective of general practice, the care of dementia is the same whatever the cause, although this may change as advances in therapy are made and as aetiological diagnosis becomes more important.

THE IMPORTANCE OF EARLY DIAGNOSIS

Although as yet effective treatment for dementia remains a hope for the future, early diagnosis is essential to minimize the incapacity produced by the disease process and to maintain the highest quality of life achievable as long as possible. There are a number of significant factors which operate in the patient's favour if early diagnosis is made and which can militate heavily against him if there is a failure to do so. The burden of this responsibility is firmly on the GP's shoulders now not only in terms of his general responsibility as point of first contact for most health care provision, but also with regard to the over 75s, under the terms of his new contractual obligations.

Intellectual ability has been shown to decline with age in the normal population, however it is probable that there is a gap between best possible rate of decline and actual decline. The gap is thought to be due principally to lack of stimulation. This is particularly marked in those suffering from sensory deprivation due to visual or hearing impairment or social isolation. The onset of dementia causes an acceleration in the declining curve but the gap between possible and actual levels of ability is also likely to widen in early dementia which goes undiagnosed. The patient's own reaction to his symptoms and the reactions of others, lacking knowledge of the diagnosis, may lead to increased social isolation, sensory deprivation and an unnecessarily accelerated decline.

It is during the early stages of dementia that awareness of his own declining ability produces the greatest stress on the patient, and when counselling and support are of most value. Later, lack of awareness produces some protection and these stresses are fully on the carers. Psychological and behavioural changes may reflect an individual's attempts to cope with or deny his decline, rather than the illness itself and can only be understood if the diagnosis has been made. Two parallel coping processes have been described (Leventhal *et al.*, 1984). The first is coping with the disease symptoms and the second is coping with the patient's own emotional reactions to the disease. An individual's approach will be determined by any previous knowledge which he has of the condition, especially experience amongst family and friends, by his own personality and by his perceived reactions of those around him. A depressive reaction is common, as are withdrawal and denial. Clearly, a GP, who has some knowledge of the patient and his family, is in the best position to unravel these problems and provide positive and appropriate help for the individual during these devastating initial stages of the disease.

Early diagnosis, unwelcome though it may be, can bring understanding and even relief to a perplexed and confused family. The effects of early dementia on family members has been well described by Barnes *et al.* (1981). Early subtle changes can lead to uncertainty within the family. Personality changes, such as irritability, restriction of activities and even reactive depression on the part of the patient can be misinterpreted as spiteful or wilful behaviour. Families may react to the change in the patient with a variety of emotional responses. There may be anger, withdrawal or denial with attribution of the changes to other less emotionally painful causes, such as deafness, poor sight or the normal decline of old age. If diagnosis is delayed, or there is a failure to impart it to the family, relationships within the family are more likely to deteriorate and the previously fertile ground in which to develop a caring support system at home may be tainted with guilt, resentment and confusion. This period of coming to terms with the diagnosis is one of great stress for the family and patience and understanding are the clinical skills required. Uncertainty as to what the future holds adds considerably to the problem and the GP can alleviate this by discussing the future in realistic terms whilst making clear his own continued support as well as the services available to fill present and future needs. Alzheimer's disease presents a particular problem in this respect as it may run a slow course, as is more often the pattern in late onset cases, or a rapidly progressive one with an early fatal outcome.

THE DIAGNOSIS—ITS DIFFICULTIES AND HOW GOOD ARE WE AT MAKING IT?

Dementia is defined as a constellation of signs and symptoms reflecting global impairment of higher intellectual functions. The clinical picture which

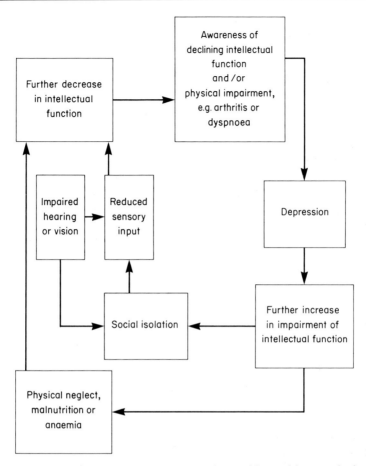

Figure 2. Cycle of interactive causes in elderly patients with or without early dementia.

may suggest progressive dementia may also have numerous other causes and combinations of causes in the elderly. The primary task is to ensure that no reversible or treatable cause is present alone or in combination with dementia. The presentation of early dementia is often precipitated by an additional treatable problem. Progressive dementia as with any diagnosis in the elderly needs to be approached cautiously, as multiple pathology is more often present and presenting symptoms can be atypical. Many problems can overlap and interweave producing a more blurred picture of disease than that found in the young. Interactions between social and physical problems are also more common with advancing age and can affect both presentation and prognosis dramatically (Fig. 2). This is well illustrated by one common example, i.e. depression. This commonly accompanies early symptoms of

Table 2. Differential diagnoses in the confused
elderly patient.

Subdural haematoma
Neurosyphilis
Parkinsonism
Low pressure hydrocephalus
Drug side effects
Hypothyroidism
Vitamin B_{12} deficiency
Alcohol, either acute confusion or dementia
Functional psychiatric disorder especially depression
Acute confusional states

dementia, and equally early symptoms of many other diseases in the elderly and also commonly occurs alone.

This cycle can occur whether a true early dementia is present or not. Even if it is, at presentation and during the early stage of the disease, a large part of the reduction in mental capacity can be due to the functional component, which is only later superseded by the effects of actual organic deterioration.

In one study of 200 cases of dementia (Smith and Hiloh, 1981), a potentially reversible cause was found in 13 patients, although these were predominantly in the under 65 age group. Table 2 illustrates not only alternative diagnoses but additional diagnoses which may contribute to the presenting symptomatology.

Clearly investigation must be designed to meet individual need and will be considered in the light of the severity of the condition and the social situation of the patient. However, taking into account the fact that any change in environment is likely to be disturbing and to cause deterioration, investigation from a home base is often preferable. Many investigations can be carried out without the necessity for hospital admission, and these are illustrated in Table 3.

Having excluded other causes or having diagnosed and treated possible causes without marked improvement of mental function, a more positive diagnosis of dementia must be made. In the UK, certainly in general practice, diagnosis is made on the basis of interview and examination and high tech investigations showing anatomical and physiological changes in the brain play little or no part at present. The wide variability of health status within the elderly population and the wide variation in performance of individuals with the same chronological age makes any assessment difficult. The individual's state of mental functioning and decline can only be predicted and assessed at any particular age in the broadest terms by comparison with statistical averages. However, there are physiological and psychological changes associated with ageing which provide benchmarks against which organic changes can be assessed (Schneider and Rowe, 1990).

Table 3. Investigations open to general practitioners
without hospital admission.

- Biochemistry
  U and E
  Liver function
  Bone chemistry
  Plasma glucose

- Haematology
  FBC
  ESR
  B_{12} and folate levels

- Thyroid function tests

- Syphilis serology

- Chest and skull X-rays

- MSU

- Other specific investigations suggested by individual history

As dementia is a global impairment of intellectual ability it is necessary to assess a number of variables, i.e. not just memory loss. Any screening test used in general practice must be simple enough to administer with only a brief training and must be acceptable to the elderly people to whom it is given, some of whom will not be suffering from dementia. It must however correlate well with the more complex tests and produce consistent assessment results in the hands of different practitioners. The development of dementia, though variable in rate between individuals, is really a continuum of impairment. Tests are essential both to define an agreed point at which it is accepted that dementia has been reached and in order to consistently describe degrees of severity.

The confused elderly patient is in a vulnerable state and a change of environment can intefere with assessment. Scores go down for any test administered outside the home and these reductions are more marked when testing is done after acute admission to hospital following a crisis at home. Clearly the GP or community nurse are the personnel most ideally suited to this task. There are many tests available, some extremely complex, however fortunately there are simple tests which have been found to be reliable. Two tests which are widely used are the Mini-Mental State Examination (MMSE) as described by Folstein *et al.* (1975) and the Clifton Assessment Procedures for the Elderly (CAPE) (Pattie and Gilleard, 1979). The MMSE takes only 10 min but detects close to 90% of dementia and delirium cases (Anthony *et al.*, 1982). CAPE has two parts. The first part is similar to MMSE and the second part is a behaviour rating scale filled out by a nurse, relative or someone familiar with the patient in his home environment. Despite the fact that these two tests are screening instruments and not full assessments, they

Table 4. Areas of cognitive function and social performance assessed in the Clinical Dementia Rating (CDR).

- Memory
- Orientation
- Judgement
- Problem solving
- Participation in community affairs
- Life at home and hobbies
- Personal care

Reproduced with permission, from Hughes *et al.* (1982).

provide easily obtained invaluable information. The Clinical Dementia Rating is also a useful scale which places people along a continuum from health to severe dementia by assessing each of the areas shown in Table 4 (Hughes *et al.*, 1982). Data of this type provide a baseline from which the rate of decline can be measured and predictions, as far as ever possible, can be made. They allow more accurate planning for provision of care and for realistic discussion of the future with relatives.

If early diagnosis is important, albeit difficult, the question which must be asked is, 'How good are GPs at doing this and are we improving?'. In Williamson's study of the unreported needs of elderly people he found that four out of five cases of dementia which they diagnosed during home interviews were unrecognized by the family physician (Williamson *et al.*, 1964). In 1988 O'Connor *et al.* studied seven practices in Cambridge and asked GPs to place a group of patients into one of three categories:

- definitely not demented,
- possibly demented, or
- definitely demented.

When compared with independent assessments, GPs were only correct in 58% of all cases. They were only correct in 65% of those who had moderate or severe dementia. Perhaps even more disturbing was a group of 20% of the patients who were incorrectly diagnosed as demented but who in fact suffered from functional psychiatric disorders, mainly depression. Unfortunately these rather unsatisfactory figures were confirmed in 1991 by Iliffe *et al.* who found similar numbers. In the O'Connor study community nurses were also assessed, albeit on a smaller number of patients. They correctly identified 86% of all cases and 96% of those with moderate or severe dementia. They did however mis-classify more patients as demented who in fact had functional problems. Two clear messages emerge from these data. The first is well known to all practising GPs and the above data merely serve to illustrate it, i.e. the community nurse is an invaluable asset. The second is that GP education in this area is woefully inadequate and seems not to have improved in recent years. One of the accepted reasons why early clear diagnosis is important is to enable the GP to prepare the family appropriately. Even when a correct diagnosis has been made it is little use if it remains within the notes and the doctor's mind, so a useful rider is the question 'How good are GPs as a group at communicating the diagnosis and prognosis and thus preparing the family for what is to come?'. One study based on the views and wishes of carers themselves suggested that information was given far too late, if ever (Morgan, 1989).

MANAGEMENT

Our policy of caring for the chronically sick, including the patient with dementia, within the community is not the case throughout Europe. For example, Denmark and The Netherlands favour institutional care, but in Italy and Spain community care is preferred. The step-wise deterioration which occurs when patients enter institutional care strongly suggests that home care is to the patient's advantage. Thus, from the GP's point of view diagnosis is only the beginning and the foundation upon which continuing care is based. The GP who has made and communicated the diagnosis is often the most suitable person to take on the case, and may already find himself in a position of trust within the family. It is important that once this responsibility has been accepted by a particular GP, he should not at any time withdraw.

The frequency of his contact may vary considerably depending on the rate of change in individual cases and other support available, but his constant involvement and availability must be known to the patient and family. As the disease progresses the practical, psychological and social needs of the patient and his carers will change and having been identified at the outset will require constant monitoring and adjustment.

The management of a patient with dementia within the community can be artificially but usefully divided into two overlapping areas, i.e. care for the patient himself and care for the carers. This avoids the pitfall of transferring all attention to supporting the carers, once the management structure has been set up. Both patient and carers require consideration of their practical, psychological and social needs.

The patient

There is a danger, once dementia is moderate and communication with the patient himself becomes difficult, of assessing his needs only through the carers. This can lead to unnecessary suffering due to problems which the patient cannot express and of which the carers either are unaware or assume are an inevitable consequence of the disease. The general principles of care in the elderly should not be forgotten, as problems which are common in the elderly are just as common in the elderly with dementia. The control of ongoing symptoms and newly appearing symptoms unrelated or only peripherally related to dementia is only possible if the patient is closely observed and examined periodically. A few common conditions in the elderly deserve mention and serve to illustrate this point. The distressing dyspnoea of incipient congestive cardiac failure, especially nocturnal dyspnoea, and the increasing pain of worsening arthritis can be easily missed. Malnutrition and anaemia should be looked for specifically. A Department of Social Security survey of the elderly showed that the prevalence of malnutrition rose with age. In the over 70s, 12% of men and 8% of women were malnourished. Confusion and depression as well as ill fitting or painful dentures were found to be important factors. Vision and hearing should not be ignored especially in early and moderate dementia. This is not only because of the possible acceleration in decline which can result from sensory deprivation, but because of the comfort which can come from watching TV or listening to a radio, even with reduced comprehension. Any suggestion of depression should be treated because of its contribution to reduced cognitive function, and also because of the added distress which it may be causing. However, it must be remembered that the usefulness of this treatment, as all others, should be constantly monitored. A point may be reached when stopping treatment may be as beneficial as starting it had been.

The distress caused to both patients and carers by other more obvious practical problems can often be reduced considerably by advice from the GP or advice and simple training by skilled community nurses. Constipation due to immobility can be controlled with dietary supplements or treated with medication. Later on faecal incontinence may need to be approached by controlled doses of a constipating agent like codeine phosphate with nursing care in using suppositories, enemas or even manual extraction to prevent discomfort. Likewise incontinence of urine can be less distressing for both patient and carers if regular bladder emptying is practised, and it is sometimes possible to achieve an established routine with the help of good nursing advice, education and encouragement. It is said by some that nocturnal incontinence due to the use of hypnotics can be improved by changing to a shorter acting compound. This can be tried but is another example of a change which should be monitored carefully, as the increased nocturnal wandering and disturbance which may follow can be more troublesome and dangerous than the wet bed.

The psychological needs of the patient stressed by the dawning awareness of his condition have been discussed, and these needs continue until awareness recedes. The use of psychotherapy is dismissed by many in the early stages of dementia. However, clinical observations suggest that not only do some patients have insight but also welcome the opportunity to discuss their distress (Reisberg *et al.*, 1982). Reminiscence therapy, where such aids as photographs or music are used to stimulate discussion and evoke memories of pleasing past events, has been little assessed but has been found rewarding by formal and informal carers alike (Jaques, 1988).

Caring for the carers

Demographic changes have led to the elderly nowadays having fewer children who live further away then they used to. Middle-aged women, the traditional carers, are now more often working as well as raising a family, and trends show an increasing number of men and the elderly as carers. One study showed that 37% of carers of the demented were over 70 years, and the average age was 61 years (Levin, 1983). A study in 1983 focused on the problems faced by carers and four main problem areas emerged (Table 5) (Levin, 1983). These were confirmed as being the areas of most problem by O'Connor *et al.* (1990).

Almost all patients with dementia will need some practical assistance as soon as a diagnosis has been reached and may already be in receipt of some services. However as the disease progresses they will need continual supervision and attention throughout the day and night. The point will be reached when they must be helped to get up, washed, fed, dressed and put to bed, and during the course of the day supervised in order to prevent them damaging themselves or property. The stress of this burden alone is immense. The GP as family physician will probably know or have as patients on his list the informal carers carrying this burden, and is likely to be the person to whom requests for help are first made. As the disease progresses anticipation of increasing needs before a breaking point is reached can allow community care to continue effectively for longer. The services which are theoretically

Table 5. Four main problem areas faced by carers.

- **Practical**—giving the elderly person regular help with household and personal care, for example, getting their relatives up, washed and dressed, toileting them, making sure they ate, putting them to bed.

- **Behaviour of the elderly person**—for example, incontinence, repetitive questions, aggression, wandering, unsafe acts, night disturbance.

- **Interpersonal**—for example, sadness at the change in their relatives, losing their tempers with them and tension in their households.

- **Social**—for example, restrictions on getting out, seeing family and friends, having a holiday, going out to work.

Reproduced with permission, from Levin *et al.* (1983).

Table 6. Main types of domiciliary support services available.

Supplier	Service
Local authority social services	Social workers Home helps Meals on wheels Family aides Night sitters Foster care Day centres (and transport) Financial assistance Relief admissions Carers' support groups

National Health Service	District Nurse/health visitor
	Physiotherapist[a]
	Occupational therapist[a]
	Community psychiatric nurse
	Nurse continence adviser
	Incontinence laundry service
	Incontinence aids
	Aids for: walking
	          toileting
	          hearing
	          vision
	Wheelchairs, prostheses
	Dental services
	Day hospitals (and transport)
	Relief admissions
	Carers' support groups

Voluntary agencies	Carers' support groups Transport Day centres Social events Foster care Assorted help schemes, e.g. sitting, gardening
Private sector	A growing variety of home support services are becoming available

[a]Sometimes provided by social services
Reproduced with permission, from Byrne and Arie (1990).

available to assist are shown in Table 6. Many of these are aimed at carer support, but how effective are they?

Setting aside the question of whether the total amount of resources available is adequate or not, there is evidence that those available are deployed in an uncoordinated fashion and that there is much duplication, inappropriate use and falling between stools. Another problem is the marked regional variation in types of service, their quality and the quantum available. The GP is ideally placed to know which resources are most readily available in his area, how pressed they are and consequently when and where to use them appropriately without waste. One study found that most effort was spent in Britain supporting the demented patient living alone in the community, even though ultimately the situation was rarely viable (Bergmann *et al.*, 1978). It was their view that services would be better directed at patients with family support. Little attention seems to have been paid to this view. A study in 1990 which studied services provided particularly with the carer in mind showed that households where there is a carer present tend to be selected against regarding provision of social services involving help with personal domestic care (Twigg *et al.*, 1990). This seems to be the case despite the fact that, in a comprehensive study of carers in 1983, home help was one of the particularly highly valued services (Levin *et al.*, 1983).

Even where services are available, the quantum is often too low and many are available only intermittently. District nurses can provide a range of practical services for example bathing (though less in recent years), changing dressings, administering medication and advising and supporting carers. Twilight nursing services are particularly valuable but are only available in some areas, and then are highly stressed by demand. Social services are likely to be a linchpin in terms of supporting carers and these are coordinated by and in the control of the social worker. Sadly the local availability of services and the attitudes and behaviour of those providing them vary enormously. They are generally inflexible and therefore unable to respond to immediate and unplanned needs. Respite care, whether on a full-time periodic basis or on a regular day care basis, is greatly appreciated by carers. Sometimes it is requested by carers but some need encouragement to accept it, yet the break from the burden of caring, both physical and emotional, can revive a caring situation which might otherwise break down. A local knowledge of resources is necessary to fit individual carer's needs, as respite care can be arranged with voluntary group sitters, local authority day care centres and temporary beds in residential homes or hospital beds. Despite the fact that some dementia patients receive many different types of support, these often do not match their needs or the needs of their principal carers. One of the obstacles to the delivery of appropriate services is the historical division between health and social services. The voluntary agencies who fill vital areas of need not provided for by government, or prop up the services which are provided but inadequate, are often working in isolation. Indeed, in the new world of supply and purchase within the NHS they may well be placed in the ridiculous position of being in competition with each other for care funding. However, this bleak picture is relieved by many encouraging local examples of collaboration based on multidisciplinary teams. In Lewisham the Community team for Mental Health in the elderly can be contacted by GPs, relatives or friends. In Bradford a general practice based scheme formally involves voluntary organizations.

The Levin study (1983) described two aspects of the psychological stress suffered by carers, i.e. that of coping with the behaviour of the patient and the interpersonal problems which arise such as sadness or anger. Behaviour problems illustrate well the two-fold burden which the carer has to bear. Common behaviour problems such as incontinence, repetitive questioning, aggression, wandering, unsafe acts and night disturbance impose both a practical burden and the emotional one of watching a loved one turn into an unrecognizable stranger. A study by Greene *et al.* (1982) described two types of behaviour which relatives find most difficult to cope with. The first is passive withdrawn behaviour which leads to feelings of rejection within the family. The carers became depressed and felt that their own health was suffering. The second was unstable mood. Angry, aggressive, accusing or moody behaviour on the part of the patient produced a negative response leaving carers feeling embarrassed, angry and frustrated. It is noteworthy that these problems seemed more important than the patient's inability to perform everyday self care skills.

The GP's role in helping the carers and the whole family to cope with these feelings of sadness, guilt and loss which are evoked is two-fold. Early preparation in advance of the progress of the disease can help significantly to alleviate distress (Wilcock *et al.*, 1991). Table 7 suggests a list of useful points for relatives. It provides a combination of practical advice with a reminder of the emotional problems which must be faced by the GP and the family, and which are all too easy to avoid. Individual carers obviously require a sympathetic approach tailored to their own needs and personality, but open discussion of the fact that the loved one no longer exists and has been replaced by the person you are caring for can both defuse tension and relieve stress. In my experience the penultimate piece of advice is particularly important, i.e. prepare yourself psychologically for the day when he no longer recognizes you. However aware the carer is of the patient's limited cognitive function, the point at which the patient no longer recognizes him is still an extremely difficult emotional hurdle, and feelings of rejection evoked by it may lead to a breakdown in caring. Gentle preparation and discussion in advance are invaluable. If care within the family is to be maintained, the social needs of the carers and their families must not be forgotten. In their 1981 study of carers, Barnes *et al.* described the time required as dementia progressed as a major stress factor. The time and energy involved in some cases became so overwhelming that carers often lost sight of their own personal needs and interests and their relationship with other family members. Loss of employment or loss of job opportunity by a carer, physical or emotional neglect of other members of the family, and social isolation are common problems. Tensions and resentments can develop within a family which increase the stress of the primary carer. Intervention at a counselling or psychotherapeutic level may be necessary as may be an

Table 7. Useful points for relatives.

- Alzheimer's disease is a terminal illness. Nobody ever gets better from it. Most are dead within 7 years.
- It is good to start grieving for the loss of the demented person now. The person who you knew, for example as your parent or spouse, now no longer exists, but has been replaced by the person you now care for.
- Take every opportunity you can to talk about your predicament with other people in the same position. This is often just as useful as talking to professionals. The Alzheimer's Disease Society exists to put you in touch (UK phone number: 081 675 6557).
- Accept an offer of day care for your relative. It will give you much-needed respite from the task of looking after your relative.
- Lock up any rooms in the house which you do not use. Your relative will not notice this restriction, and this may make your life much easier.
- Lock any drawers which contain important papers or easily-spoiled items. This will prevent the patient storing inappropriate things in them, such as compost from the garden, or worse.
- Remove locks from the lavatory so he cannot get locked in.
- Normal sexual relationships will probably stop. Spouses should try not to fall into the trap of asking 'What's the matter with me?'
- Prepare yourself psychologically for the day when he no longer recognizes you. This can be a great blow, unless you prepare for it.
- Apply to Social Services for an Attendance Allowance, if appropriate.

Note: we do not envisage giving such stark advice to the carer the moment the diagnosis is made. Some groundwork needs to be done first. However, all the evidence (based on the wishes of the carers themselves) is that we tend to give this sort of advice far too late, if ever (Morgan, 1989). Reproduced with permission, from Wilcock *et al.* (1991).

increase in practical help and/or respite care to maintain the caring unit as a viable one. Early intervention, before a crisis point has been reached is always best, but this can only be achieved if a sensitive and consistent monitoring role has been maintained by the GP.

The value of carers' and relatives' support groups run by voluntary organizations and local authorities should be mentioned. They both deal with problems in a practical, problem-solving way and allow carers to explore and share the complex emotional and social problems which they face. A GP's local knowledge of such groups, and encouragement of carers to attend despite the pressures on their time, is important.

Breaking point—the need for institutional care

Even the most devoted carer may reach a breaking point at which he feels unable to go on. When all other available help has been tapped it is the duty of the GP to broach the question of institutional care. Indeed, it is necessary to be alert to the warning signals of this situation approaching as an overall balance of cost to the carers and benefit to the patient must be drawn. Abuse of the elderly is an increasingly recognized problem. Research shows that unrelenting stress is the chief factor associated with abuse, so the elderly patient with dementia must be one of the most vulnerable. Carers have expressed immense relief when asked about their feelings of aggression. From the carer's point of view tensions created within a family may lead to severe health problems for one member, or even the breakdown of a family unit with incalculable consequences. Sometimes the picture is one of gradual increase in strain with time and the deterioration in the patient's condition. Alternatively there may be a sudden alteration in the carer's tolerance and ability to cope due to an extraneous event, for example sickness in another relative or an acute financial problem necessitating the primary carer's return to work. The delicate balancing of the patient's rights and wishes if ascertainable and the multiple potential risks to the well being of carers and others is an ethical minefield. The GP is usually involved in the decision as to when and where the patient should be admitted and his help is usually sought in making arrangements. The patient with dementia is entirely incapable of weighing up any information which he may be given, and the GP needs to keep a clear head in assessing, as best he can, the needs of the patient and his carers. Solutions are best arrived at when they are made in calm not crisis, and with the advice and involvement of all those involved with the care of the patient, that is to say informal and formal carers. Even if the outcome is the same, relatives and close carers often suffer psychologically later if sudden decisions are come to in a crisis situation. Temporary respite care can allow time for a calm decision to be arrived at to avert this unsatisfactory conclusion. The elderly patient with dementia living alone poses different but equally difficult ethical problems. He may be considered by relatives or neighbours incapable of making informed decisions, and pressure is brought upon the GP to 'do something,' as the patient is considered to be a danger to himself and others. This paternalistic view has some merits and the anxieties of those expressing it are often genuine. However, there is the opposing view that the patient who lives happily alone, even for a shorter time, is better off than one living unhappily in an institution.

CONCLUSION

It would seem clear that in the future better provision for patients with dementia within the community necessitates better GP education in the area of diagnosis and recognition, as well as better coordination of community support services. Once the management structure has been set up, the GP's role is both to monitor closely changing needs and to identify new ones. This cannot be done effectively from behind a bank of computer terminals, valuable though modern technology is, but by regularly visiting the home and giving time to the patient and his carers.

REFERENCES

Anthony, J.C., Le Resche, L., Niaz, U., Von Horff, M.R. and Folstein, M.F. (1982). Limits of the 'Mini Mental State' as a screening test for dementia and delirium among hospital patients. *Psychol. Med.*, **12**, 397–408.

Barnes, R.F., Raskind, M.A., Scott, M. and Murphy, C. (1981). Problems of families caring for Alzheimer patients: use of a support group. *J. Am. Geriatr. Soc.*, **29**, 80–85.

Bergmann, K., Foster, E.M., Justic, A.W. and Matthews, V. (1978). Management of the demented elderly patient in the community. *Br. J. Psychiatry*, **132**, 441–449.

Byrne, E.J. and Arie, T. (1990). Coping with dementia in the elderly. In: Lawson, D.H. (Ed.), *Current Medicine—2*. Churchill Livingstone, Edinburgh.

Copeland, J.R.M. (1990). Epidemiological aspects of the mental disorders of old age. In: Bergener, Ermini and Stakelin (Eds), *Challenges in Aging*. Academic Press, London.

Folstein, M.F., Folstein, S.E. and McHugh, P.R. (1975). 'Mini Mental State': a practical method for grading the cognitive state of patients for the clinician. *J. Psychiatr. Res.*, **12**, 189–198.

Greene, J.G., Smith, R., Gardiner, M. and Timbury, G.C. (1992). Measuring behavioural disturbance of elderly demented patients in the community and its effect on relatives: a factor analytic study. *Age Ageing*, **11**, 121–126.

Hughes, C.P., Berg, L., Danziger, W.L., Coben, L.A. and Martin, R.L. (1982). A new clinical scale for the staging of dementia. *Br. J. Psychiatry*, **140**, 566–567.

Iliffe, S., *et al.* (1991). Assessment of elderly people in general practice: social circumstances and mental stage. *Br. J. Gen. Pract.*, **41**, 9–12.

Ineichen, B. (1987). Measuring the rising tide: how many dementia carers will there be by 2001? *Br. J. Psychiatry*, **150**, 193–200.

Jaques, A. (1988). *Understanding Dementia*. Churchill Livingstone, Edinburgh.

Laing, W. and Hall, M. (1991). The challenge of aging. In: Lumley, P. (Ed.), *Agenda for Health*, Association of the British Pharmaceutical Industry, London.

Leventhal, H., Nerenz, D.R. and Steele, D.J. (1984). Illness representations and coping with health threats. In: Baum, A., Taylor, S.E. and Singel, S.E. (Eds), *Handbook of Health Psychology, Vol. IV*.

Levin, E. (1983). The elderly and their informal carers. In: Allen, I., Levin, E., Sidell, M. and Vetter, N. (Eds), *Research Contributions to the Development of Policy and Practice*. HMSO, London, pp. 69–91.

Levin, E., Sinclair, I. and Gorbach, P. (1983). *The Supporters of Confused Elderly Persons at Home*. National Institute for Social Work, London.

Levin, E., Sinclair, I. and Gorbach, P. (1989). *Families, Services and Confusion in Old Age*. Gower, Aldershot.

Morgan, M.J. (1989). Looking after a patient with Alzheimer's disease. *Br. Med. J.*, **299**, 1606–1607.

O'Connor, D.W. *et al.* (1988). Do general practitioners miss dementia in elderly patients? *Br. Med. J.*, **297**, 1107–1110.

O'Connor, D.W. *et al.* (1989). The prevalence of dementia as measured by the Cambridge mental disorders of the elderly examination. *Acta Psychiatr. Scand.*, **79**, 190–198.

O'Connor, D.W. *et al.* (1990). Problems reported by relatives in a community study of dementia. *Br. J. Psychiatry*, **156**, 835–841.

Pattie, A.H. and Gilleard, C.J. (1979). *Manual of the Clifton Assessment Procedures for the Elderly (CAPE)*. Hodder & Stoughton, Sevenoaks.

Reisberg, B., Ferris, S.H., de Leon, M.J. and Crook, T. (1982). The global deterioration scale for assessment of primary degenerative dementia. *Am. J. Psychiatry*, **139**, 1136–1139.

Schneider, E.L. and Rowe, J.W. (1990). *Handbook of the Biology of Aging.* Academic Press, London.

Smith, J.S. and Hiloh, L.G. (1981). The investigation of dementia: results in 200 consecutive admissions. *Lancet*, **i**, 824–827.

Twigg, J., Atkin, K. and Perring, C. (1990). *Carers and Services: A Review of Research.* HMSO, London.

Wilcock, G.K., Gray, J.A.M. and Longmore, J.M. (1991). *Geriatric Problems in General Practice, 2nd edn.* Oxford University Press, Oxford.

Williamson, J., Stokoe, I.H., Gray, M.S., Fisher, M., Smith, A., McGhee, A. and Stephenson, E. (1964). Old people at home: their unreported needs. *Lancet*, **i**, 1117–1120.

7

Drug Therapy in Relation to Current Knowledge

MICHAEL FRASER SHANKS

Consultant Psychiatrist, Highland Health Board and Honorary Senior Lecturer, Aberdeen University, UK

INTRODUCTION

There is an urgent need to improve the treatment of behavioural disturbances seen in the course of Alzheimer's disease and other dementias, but progress and understanding in this respect offer a poor contrast with the intense activity and developing understanding at a molecular level. It is the behavioural disturbances, often episodic, which lead to medical and social crises and stress relatives and staff, the latter increasingly in non-hospital settings (Rabins, 1990). Disturbed behaviour is particularly associated with the complication of delirium, and here medical assessment and investigation to determine cause, for example anaemia, hypothyroidism or infection, is essential. Episodic or persistent delirium may appear however in the course of the natural history of dementia, when it cannot be readily linked to a definable systemic illness (Perry *et al.*, 1990). Behavioural problems appear as disturbances of the sleep/wake cycle, delusions, hallucinations, and disinhibition including aggression and wandering. Sometimes an emotional disorder complicates the dementing process, with syndromes of depressive illness or anxiety states (Burns *et al.*, 1990). Psychotropic drugs or drugs given for other conditions may themselves contribute to cognitive and emotional changes (Larson *et al.*, 1987; Emerich and Sanberg, 1991), while environmental factors strongly influence behaviour in the dementias.

The possible remedies available to the clinician are those of the battlefield surgeon! Psychotropic treatment is in any case rarely based on a substantial understanding of the pathophysiology and in the dementias investigation of natural history, nosology and neurochemistry are still at an early stage. Drugs interact with a nervous system already substantially damaged and with demonstrable deficits in several neurotransmitter systems (Bowen, 1990). Add to this the well known extra hazards of drug treatment even in normal elderly subjects (Ouslander, 1981), and the idiosyncracies of brain function at the molecular level (Van Tol *et al.*, 1992) and the limitations and vagaries of drug responses in individual patients come as no surprise. Accurate diagnostic information together with the general principles of good prescribing practice (and perhaps an understanding of the psychodynamics of prescribing) can however often mitigate behavioural problems without causing unacceptable side effects.

MAJOR TRANQUILLIZERS IN AGITATION AND PSYCHOSIS

The excessive prescription of these drugs for dementia sufferers has drawn comment for many years (Barton and Hurst, 1966; Gilleard *et al.*, 1983), and recent American studies highlight a problem that very likely continues to exist in this country as well (Beers *et al.*, 1988; Avorn *et al.*, 1992). Avorn *et al.* reported a randomized controlled trial of psychotropic drug reduction or withdrawal in a nursing home setting. There was no increase in measures of behavioural disturbance or staff distress. The patients from whom antipsychotics were withdrawn showed less deterioration in some aspects of cognition at follow-up, but were more likely to self report 'depression'. Two well designed placebo controlled studies tried to address whether antipsychotic drugs are actually effective in controlling agitation and other disturbed behaviours (Barnes *et al.*, 1982; Petrie *et al.*, 1982). There were only modest advantages in a few patients and placebo preparations were often as useful. The dosages of antipsychotics (loxapine, thioridazine, haloperidol) were high compared with UK practices and adverse effects in the treatment groups were marked. Favourable responses were seen in some cases with agitation, excitement, hallucinations, hostility and suspicion but not with repetitive pacing or calling activities. One antipsychotic was as good (or as bad) as another. Few investigations address specifically the efficacy of antipsychotics in controlling symptoms of the psychoses which may herald or accompany the diagnosis of dementia. It is often asserted that antipsychotics will be as effective in these schizophreniform disturbances of old age as in younger subjects, but such statements are usually based on clinical practice rather than reliable clinical trial data. It is important to distinguish suspicion and paranoid thinking based on memory disturbance and disorientation from psychotic thinking fuelled by abnormal experiences. Side effects may mean that in individual patients an antipsychotic effect cannot be attained without undue risk, although Phanjoo and Link (1990) reported advantages of remoxipride over thioridazine.

In practice, antipsychotic drugs with prominent muscarinic receptor-blocking activity (e.g. chlorpromazine, thioridazine) do not seem to cause more cognitive impairment at least in sensible dosage. Orthostatic hypotension can also be avoided by using low doses. This side effect can appear with haloperidol as well, and this drug is also more likely to cause akathisic motor disturbances, pseudoparkinsonism and late-onset dyskinesias. Many prescribers still do not appreciate the potency of haloperidol (nearly 50 times that of thioridazine). Akathisia may be difficult to distinguish from the behaviour which prompted the prescription in the first place. Elderly patients are particularly sensitive to the extrapyramidal side effects of major tranquillizers, and distinctive neuropathological changes may render some patients liable to severe and persistent neurotoxic reactions, as well as the more extreme extrapyramidal side effects (McKeith et al., 1992). Neuroleptic malignant syndromes may be under reported in the elderly with all types of dementia (Adozzonizio, 1991).

In general only a small group of patients will benefit and then only for a short time. Treatment should have identifiable goals and be regularly reviewed. The drug should be withdrawn if ineffective and in any case after a period of prescription as the problem may have remitted. Starting doses should be haloperidol 0.25 mg or thioridazine 10 mg given up to four times daily. Rarely, depot fluspirilene or other depot neuroleptics may be preferred if compliance is an issue, and here again dosage should be minimal. Injected shorter acting preparations are more potent than oral drugs, and dosage should be adjusted accordingly. Eimer (1989) offers a useful review of prescribing and side effects. The side effect profile may dictate a change of preparation for a particular patient, but in general with low dosage there is little to choose between the different groups of antipsychotic drugs.

OTHER DRUGS FOR AGITATION

There are a few studies and reports of useful suppression of agitation and related behaviour by drugs which are not major tranquillizers. Gleason and Schneider (1990) in a carbamazepine study which was not placebo controlled or blinded found improvements in agitation and hostility in five of nine outpatients with probable Alzheimer's disease. All had failed to respond to thioridazine and/or haloperidol but unfortunately the dosages and details of the withdrawal process from these drugs are not given. Dosages were increased until carbamazepine levels thought to be therapeutic in epileptic disorders were achieved. There is no assessment of depressive symptoms, although two patients had failed to respond to trazodone. The significance of this finding is uncertain, but the time course of improvement does suggest a specific drug effect.

Two Lancet letters (O'Neil et al., 1986; Greenwald et al., 1986) refer to modification of aggressive behaviours in single patients with mental impairment and dementia using a combination of trazodone and L-tryptophan to enhance central serotonin activity. Simpson and Foster (1986) report four cases with severe behaviour disturbance responding to trazodone 200–500 mg used alone or in combination with their other medication, and these patients had not responded to other antidepressants. These reports have not so far led to controlled trials, although they add weight to the clinical impression that empirical trials of antidepressant drugs should be undertaken in such cases.

Another *Lancet* letter (Petrie and Ban, 1981) described a favourable response of disturbed behaviour in three patients with dementia when propranolol was substituted in doses of 60–160 mg daily for what appear very high doses of major tranquillizers. Yudofsky *et al.* (1981) offer another, but again rather anecdotal report of the efficacy of propranolol. Greendyke and Kanter (1986) in a double-blind controlled study found that hostility and repetitive behaviours in a group of non-Alzheimer patients with severe organic brain disease favourably responded to pindolol 40–60 mg daily. It would seem that beta-blockers too might be worth a try *in extremis*, with careful monitoring of heart rate and blood pressure.

DEPRESSIVE AND ANXIETY DISORDERS

Anxious and depressive symptoms are more prominent in those with less cognitive deficit (Burns *et al.*, 1990) and therefore in the earlier stages of the illness, but emotional disorder can appear at any time and in the later stages often presents atypically. Accurate clinical assessment and attention to the statements of staff and relatives are essential.

The anticholinergic effects of tricyclic antidepressants seem to exacerbate disturbances of cognition less than one would expect on theoretical grounds, at least at the dosages usually employed. Higher doses can cause an obvious increase in disorientation and even delirium in some patients. Studies of the treatment of depression in dementia are limited, but Katz *et al.* (1990) in an appropriately designed trial studied the relative merits of nortriptyline and placebo in a residential care setting in patients with major depression. Some of these patients had 'mild to moderate cognitive impairment'. There was a highly significant advantage for nortriptyline over placebo. In relation to efficacy, Gosselin and Anchill (1989) made the intriguing finding that commonly used doses of doxepin can in some psychogeriatric subjects result in undetectable plasma levels, and recommend monitoring of plasma levels. It is not clear whether this phenomenon is confined to doxepin, although a similar group taking desipramine did develop levels in the therapeutic range. Desipramine and nortriptyline have the least muscarinic receptor blocking activity of the tricyclics, and are perhaps to be preferred for this reason. Where tricyclics are used staff must be alert for the common side effects of constipation, retention and postural hypotension. If patients develop these side effects, then trazodone or one of the serotonin specific reuptake inhibitors may be used. Fluoxetine should be used with caution because of its long half-life and increased potential for accumulation in the elderly. Starting doses should be half of those used in younger subjects. In general, depression should be treated as vigorously as in a younger patient, including the use of combined antidepressants and monoamine oxidase inhibitors (MAOI) in appropriate cases. A trial of an MAO-B inhibitor, L-deprenyl produced favourable results in one study (Tariot et al., 1987). Trials in the non-demented elderly with depression suggest that relapse after a successful MAOI treatment is less frequent than with nortryptyline (Georgotas, 1989).

Anxiety states with panic and fearfulness frequently accompany the early stages of dementia where insight or partial insight is retained. If benzodiazepines are used for ad hoc treatment, then those with a short half-life such as oxazepam are preferred. These drugs produce less cumulative toxicity with the risk of worsening psychomotor performance, and in particular causing falls (Ray et al., 1987). In practice however, anxious mood with restlessness and insomnia in dementia sufferers is more likely to respond to antidepressant drugs or low dose major tranquillizers like thioridazine (Salzman, 1990).

SLEEP DISTURBANCE

Sleep disturbance and in particular episodic or persistent nocturnal wakefulness usually challenges carers at some stage in the progression of dementia. The exclusion of delirium or emotional disorder as causes, and the appropriate investigation and treatment of these conditions if possible is important. Many of the drugs commonly prescribed for the elderly can impair sleep (Gottlieb, 1990) and in demented patients excessive sedation during the day is often a factor. When marked and persistent polyphasic patterns of sleep/wake activity appear otherwise in the course of a dementia, then the best methods of management are often environmental rather than pharmacological. The same principles as in normal elderly subjects (Moran et al., 1988) may be applied. In institutional settings increasing stimulation during the day with sleep restriction and the avoidance of excessive sedation can reduce the need for hypnotic medication with its associated problems. There are few clinical trials of the efficacy and side effects of commonly used hypnotics in dementia populations, and they are certainly over-used (Gilleard, 1985). Reynolds et al. (1988) recommend thioridazine 25–75 mg at night where there is marked behavioural disturbance during periods of wakefulness. Otherwise, short-acting hypnotics like temazepam and chlormethiazole may be used with regular review of their indications and possible hazards in a given patient.

VASCULAR AGENTS

Vasodilators

The ergoloid mesylate Hydergine, has been very widely prescribed in dementia for nearly 40 years. Hollister and Yesavage (1984) reviewed the many studies of its efficacy up till then and concluded that most had design flaws; patient populations were mixed, doses were too small and the duration of the investigations too short. Improvements in attitude, mood and behaviour were reported without however any demonstrable advance in cognition even when appropriate measurement instruments were used. Thompson *et al.* (1990) entered 80 patients with probable Alzheimer's disease in a six month placebo-controlled trial using the recommended dose (3 mg daily) of Hydergine. Both groups showed a decline in psychometric test scores, and the Hydergine group deteriorated significantly more on some tests. The authors speculated about a toxic drug effect. On the other hand, Nicergoline, another ergot derivative, was reported to improve orientation in a third of patients entered in a six month placebo-controlled trial (Battaglia *et al.*, 1989). It would seem reasonable if such drugs are prescribed to have a baseline and follow-up psychometric assessment and cease prescribing if there is no demonstrable benefit. A variety of other drugs with vasodilator and cerebral metabolic enhancing effects have been given to demented subjects with established cerebrovascular disease. Favourable responses have been reported, but may be less due to vasodilator effects which are theoretically unlikely to improve cerebral metabolism, than effects on neurotransmitter systems with antidepressant responses (see Katona, 1989). Calcium channel blockers (e.g. nimodipine) may improve focal brain ischaemia and limit excitotoxicity. The results of clinical trials are awaited.

Antihypertensives

There is a high prevalence of both hypertension and cognitive impairment in the elderly, with a substantial overlap of the two conditions so that large epidemiological studies are required to elucidate aetiological as opposed to associative relationships between the two conditions (Davidson *et al.*, 1989; Evans *et al.*, 1989). Two such studies concluded that when appropriate account was taken of age, sex, socioeconomic status, drug treatments and alcohol use, sustained hypertension was associated with cognitive impairment (Wallace *et al.*, 1985; Farmer *et al.*, 1987). Methodological problems of these and other cross-sectional and longitudinal studies mean that a causal association between hypertension and cognitive decline in the elderly is not proven. Some of these design problems have been addressed in an Edinburgh community study of untreated elderly hypertensives (Whalley, 1992, personal communication). The data suggest an age effect, lowering the blood pressure with either bendrofluazide or captopril enhanced cognitive function in the 69–75 age cohort but not in older hypertensives. The Framingham study (Farmer et al., 1987) suggested that raised blood pressure was linked to improved psychometric test scores in subjects over 75. In the younger group, vascular changes may be more important causes of cognitive decline than the parenchymatous changes of Alzheimer's disease. There may be a case therefore to treat under 75s with hypertension and cognitive impairment.

The question can also be approached from the syndromal viewpoint, and the clinically recognized if protean entity of multi-infarct dementia has been called 'preventable senility' (Hachinski, 1992). Hypertension is the major risk factor for this disorder, but Hachinski argues for a pluralist approach to the different patient groups at risk or with established cognitive changes. Preventive measures would include pharmacological strategies such as ACE inhibitors, calcium channel blockers, aspirin (Meyer et al., 1989) and anticoagulants. At-risk groups should receive advice about diet, smoking and alcohol intake. The overlap between Alzheimer's disease and the vascular dementias, together with the prominent microvascular changes in the former which may contribute to the cognitive change by parenchymal effects (Munoz, 1991) suggest that measures to improve vasoregulation or the secondary effects of ischaemia in the brain may be of benefit in both disorders. Clinically, we are now more likely to detect dementias with significant focal brain ischaemia at an earlier stage. These may present as an episode of delirium, a visual hallucinosis or the fragmentary psychotic states of 'late paraphrenia' (Almeida et al., 1992). The widespread use of SPECT scanning in these cases, if supported by history and clinical examination, may suggest significant ischaemia in the absence of CT scan changes, and allow the application of appropriate therapies. There is a very urgent need however for accurate and well designed clinical trials to rationalize treatments.

REFERENCES

Adozzonizio, G. (1991). NMS in the elderly—an under-recognised problem. Int. J. Geriatr. Psychiatry, 6, 547–549.

Almeida, O.P., Howard, R., Forstl, H. and Levy, R. (1992). Should the diagnosis of late paraphrenia be abandoned? Psychol. Med., 22, 11–14.

Avorn, J., Soumerai, S.B., Everitt, D.E., Ross-Degnan, D., Beers, M.H., Sherman, D., Salem-Sehatz, S.R. and Fields, D. (1992). A randomized trial of a program to reduce the use of psychoactive drugs in nursing homes. N. Engl. J. Med., 327, 168–173.

Barnes, R., Veith, R., Okimoto, J., Raskind, M. and Gumbrecht, G. (1982). Efficacy of anti-psychotic medications in behaviourally disturbed dementia patients. Am. J. Psychiatry, 139, 1170–1174.

Barton, R. and Hurst, L. (1966). Unnecessary use of tranquillizers in elderly patients. Br. J. Psychiatry, 112, 989–990.

Battaglia, A., Bruni, G., Ardia, A. and Sachetti, G. (1989). Nicergoline in mild to moderate dementia—a multi-center double-blind placebo controlled study. *J. Am. Geriatr. Soc.*, **37**, 295–302.

Beers, M., Avorn, J., Soumerai, S.B., Everitt, D.E., Sherman, D. and Salem, S. (1988). Psychoactive medication use in intermediate-care facility residents. *J. Am. Med. Assoc.*, **260**, 3016–3020.

Bowen, D.M. (1990). Treatment of Alzheimer's disease, molecular pathology versus neurotransmitter based therapy. *Br. J. Psychiatry*, **157**, 327–330.

Burns, A., Jacoby, R. and Levy, R. (1990). Psychiatric phenomena in Alzheimer's disease. *Br. J. Psychiatry*, **157**, 72–94.

Davidson, R.A., Hale, W.E., Moore, M.T., May, F.E., Marks, R.G. and Stewart, R.B. (1989). Incidence of hypertension in an ambulatory elderly population. *J. Am. Geriatr. Soc.*, **37**, 861–866.

Eimer, M. (1989). Management of the behavioural symptoms associated with dementia. *Prim. Care*, **16**, 431–450.

Emerich, D.F. and Sanberg, P.R. (1991). Neuroleptic dysphoria. *Biol. Psychiatry*, **29**, 201–203.

Evans, D.A., Fenkenstein, H., Albert, M.S., Scherr, P.A., Cook, N.R., Chown, M.J., Liesi, H.E., Hennekens, C.H. and Taylor, J.C. (1989). Prevalence of Alzheimer's disease in a community population of older persons. *J. Am. Med. Assoc.*, **262**, 2551–2556.

Farmer, M.E., White, L.R., Abbot, R.D., Kittner, S.J., Kaplan, E., Wolz, M.M., Brody, J.A. and Wolf, P.A. (1987) Blood pressure and cognitive performance. *Am. J. Epidemiol.*, **126**, 1103–1114.

Georgotas, A., McCue, R. and Cooper, T.B. (1989). A placebo-controlled comparison of nortryptyline and phenelzine in maintenance therapy of elderly depressed patients. *Arch. Gen. Psychiatry*, **46**, 783–786.

Gilleard, C.J., Morgan, K. and Wade, B.E. (1983). Patterns of neuroleptic use among the institutionalised elderly. *Acta. Psychiatr. Scand.*, **68**, 419–425.

Gilleard, C.J. (1985). Hypnotic prescribing amongst residents admitted to local authority homes for the elderly. *Health Bull.*, **43**, 60–63.

Gleason, R.P. and Schneider, L.S. (1990). Carbamazepine treatment of agitation in Alzheimer's out-patients refractory to neuroleptics. *J. Clin. Psychol.*, **51**, 115–118.

Gosselin, C. and Ancill, R.J. (1989). Comparative plasma levels of doxepin and desipramine in the elderly. *Can. J. Psychiatry*, **34**, 921–924.

Gottlieb, G.L. (1990). Sleep disorders and their management. Special considerations in the elderly. *Am. J. Med.*, **88** (Suppl. 3A), 29–33.

Greendyke, R.M. and Kanter, D.R. (1986). Therapeutic effects of pindolol in behavioural disturbances associated with organic brain disease: a double blind study. *J. Clin. Psychol.*, **47**, 423–426.

Greenwald, B.S., Main, D.B. and Silverman, S.M. (1986). Serotoninergic treatment of screaming and banging in dementia (Letter). *Lancet*, **ii**, 1464.

Hachinski, V. (1992). Preventable senility: a call for action against the vascular dementia. *Lancet*, **340**, 645–648.

Hollister, L.E. and Yesavage, J. (1984). Ergoloid misylates for senile dementias: unanswered questions. *Ann. Int. Med.*, **100**, 894–898.

Katona, C.L.E. (1989). Multi-infarct dementia. In Katona, C.L.E. (Ed.), *Dementia Disorders Advances and Prospects*. Chapman and Hall, London, pp. 86–103.

Katz, I..R., Simpson, G.M., Curlik, S.M., Parmalee, P.A. and Muhly, R.N. (1990). Pharmacologic treatment of major depression for elderly patients in residential care settings. *J. Clin. Psychol.*, **51** (Suppl. 7), 41–47.

Larson, E.B., Kukull, W.A., Buchner, D. and Reifler, B.V. (1987). Adverse drug reactions associated with global cognitive impairment in elderly persons. *Ann. Int. Med.*, **107**, 169–173.

McKeith, I., Fairbairn, A., Perry, R., Thompson, P. and Perry, E. (1992). Neuroleptic sensitivity in patients with senile dementia of Lewy body type. *Br. Med. J.*, **305**, 673–678.

Meyer, J.S., Rogers, R.L., McClintic, K., Mortell, K.F. and Lotfi, J. (1989). Randomized clinical trial of daily aspirin therapy in multi-infarct dementia. *J. Am. Geriatr. Soc.*, **37**, 549–555.

Moran, M.G., Thompson, T.L. and Nies, A.S. (1988). Sleep disorders in the elderly. *Am. J. Psychiatry*, **145**, 1369–1378.

Munoz, D.G. (1991). The pathological basis of multi-infarct dementia. *Alz. Dis. Ass. Dis.*, **5**, 77–90.

O'Neil, M., Page, N., Adkins, W.N. and Eichelman, B. (1986). Tryptophan-trazodone treatment of aggressive behaviour (Letter). *Lancet*, **ii**, 859.

Ouslander, J.G. (1981). Drug therapy in the elderly. *Ann. Int.Med.*, **95**, 711–722.

Perry, R.H., Irving, D., Blessed, G., Fairbairn, A.F. and Perry, E.K. (1990). Senile dementia of the Lewy body type. A clinically and neuropathologically distinct form of Lewy body dementia in the elderly. *J. Neurol. Sci.*, **95**, 119–139.

Petrie, W.M. and Ban, T.A. (1981). Propranolol in organic agitation (Letter). *Lancet*, **i**, 324.

Petrie, W.M., Ban, T.A., Berney, S., Fujimori, M., Guy, W., Ragheb, M., Wilson, W.H. and Schaffer, J.D. (1982). Loxapine in psychogeriatrics: a placebo and standard-controlled clinical investigation. *J. Clin. Psychopharmacol*, **2**, 122–126.

Phanjoo, A.L. and Link, C. (1990). Remoxipride versus thiorizadine in elderly psychotic patients. *Acta Psychiatr. Scand.*, **82** (Suppl. 358), 181–185.

Rabins, P.V., Fitting, M.D., Eastham, J. and Zabora, J. (1990). Emotional adaptation over time in care-givers for chronically ill elderly people. *Age Ageing*, **19**, 185–190.

Ray, W.A., Griffin, M.R., Schaffner, W., Baugh, D.K. and Melton, L.J. (1987). Psychotropic drug use and the risk of hip fracture. *N. Engl. J. Med.*, **316**, 363–369.

Reynolds, C.F., III, Hoch, C.C., Stack, J. and Campbell, D. (1988). The nature and management of sleep/wake disturbance in Alzheimer's dementia. *Psychoparmacol. Bull.*, **24**, 43–48.

Salzman, C. (1990). Practical considerations in the pharmacologic treatment of depression and anxiety in the elderly. *J. Clin. Psychol.*, **51**, (Suppl. 1), 40–43.

Simpson, D.M. and Foster, D. (1986). Improvement in organically disturbed behaviour with trazodone treatment. *J. Clin. Psychol.*, **47**, 191–193.

Tariot, P.N., Cohen, R.M., Sunderland, T., Newhouse, P.A., Yount, D., Mellow, A.M., Weingartner, H., Mueller, E.A. and Murphy, D.L. (1987). L-deprenyl in Alzheimer's disease. Preliminary evidence for behavioural change with monoamine oxidase B inhibition. *Arch. Gen. Psychiatry*, **44**, 427–433.

Thompson, T.L., Filley, C.M. and Mitchell, W.D. (1990). Lack of efficacy of Hydergine in patients with Alzheimer's disease. *N. Engl. J. Med.*, **323**, 445–448.

Van Tol, H.M.M., Wu, C.M., Guan, H.-C., Ohara, K., Bunzo, J.R., Civelli, O., Kennedy, J., Seeman, P., Niznik, H.B. and Jovanovic, V. (1992). Multiple dopamine D_4 receptor variants in the human population. *Nature*, **358**, 149–152.

Wallace, R.B., Lemke, J.H., Morris, M.C., Goodenberger, M., Kohout, P., Hinrichs, J.V. (1985). Relationship of free-recall memory to hypertension in the elderly: the Iowa 65+ rural health study. *J. Chronic Dis.*, **38**, 475–481.

Yudofsky, S., Williams, D. and Gorman, J. (1981). Propranolol in the treatment of rage and violent behaviour in patients with chronic brain syndromes. *Am. J. Psychiatry*, **138**, 218–220.

8

Depression in Alzheimer's Disease: Confusing, Confounding but Treatable

R.J. ANCILL

Clinical Professor and Head, Division of Geriatric Psychiatry, Department of Psychiatry, The University of British Columbia, Vancouver, Canada

INTRODUCTION

It is hard to ignore that there is a significant level of therapeutic nihilism that occurs when physicians are asked to deal with patients with Alzheimer's disease or related disorders who present with dysfunctional behaviour. There is a tendency to fall into the trap of 'dementism' whereby a patient with a dementing disorder is presumed to have no other pathology to account for the change in function or behaviour but that it must be due to the dementia. Given this view, it then follows that the 'treatment' is to suppress the behaviour with sedative drugs, often neuroleptics or benzodiazepines. These prescribing habits have been widely reported in the literature and will often result in a further deterioration in the patient because of emergent adverse events which are not recognized as drug toxicity but are mistakenly believed to reflect a worsening of the 'dementia' (Ancill *et al.*, 1988). What is poorly understood is that the dysfunctional behaviour, especially but not necesssarily if the onset has been somewhat acute, is invariably caused by underlying disease (Ancill, 1989a). Among the more common causes of acute and subacute deterioration in patients with a dementia are delirium and depression. Cognitively impaired elderly with neurodegenerative disease are especially prone to delirium produced by psychotropic drugs although other common causes include infections and anoxic states. Depression is a frequent comorbid syndrome that occurs in patients with Alzheimer's disease with an incidence that has been reported to be as high as 57% (Liston, 1978) although more recent work has suggested an incidence around 40% (Lazarus *et al.*, 1987). It should also be recognized that many patients will present with 'the 3 Ds' of dementia, delirium and depression.

COPRESENTATION OF DEPRESSION AND DEMENTIA

It is known that patients with Alzheimer's dementia are more likely than the non-demented to have a previous history of depression that predates the onset of cognitive impairment (Agbayewa, 1986). Whether this finding implies that depression may be a prodromal syndrome of Alzheimer's disease or that both disorders share some similar genetic or psychological predisposition is not clear. However, Zweig *et al.* (1993) have reported that depression in Alzheimer's disease may be associated with a loss of noradrenergic neurones in the locus ceruleus suggesting that at least some patients with both depression and dementia have a specific neuropathology to account for this comorbidity. This comorbidity has been reported in other neurodegenerative disorders. Depression is reported to occur in 40% of patients with Parkinson's disease with at least half of these meeting the DSM-IIIR criteria for major depression (Cummings, 1992).

Although historically there has been much interest and discussion around the issue of 'pseudodementia' where the cognitive impairment is secondary to a primary depressive illness (Wells, 1979), much less attention has been paid to the copresentation of depression and dementia (Reifler, 1986) including the recognition that the depressive component represents a treatable element of the combined cognitive impairment. In a recent study of elderly inpatients, 86% of geriatric patients with depression and dementia responded to antidepressive therapy, of which 26% required ECT. Furthermore, of the patients whose depression resolved, 80% showed improvements in their Mini-Mental State scores (Ancill, 1989b). However, Murphy (1983) suggested that treating depression in the elderly was associated with a poor outcome and focused on psychosocial variables to account for this. However this view has been challenged on methodological grounds as well as with data supporting a more therapeutically optimistic and opposing position (Baldwin and Jolley, 1986). This clinical situation is further complicated by failure on behalf of the clinician to recognize depression in demented individuals or by an age-related or dementia-related therapeutic nihilism even when depression is suspected or even diagnosed (Koenig *et al.*, 1992) in the mistaken belief that it is either not treatable or not worth treating.

Emory and Oxman (1992) have put forward the notion of a continuum between depressive dementia and degenerative dementia with overlapping pathophysiological mechanisms rather than differential diagnoses and this may lead to a better understanding of the copresentation of cognitive impairment and mood disorders.

RECOGNITION OF DEPRESSION IN DEMENTIA

Perhaps the major problem in addressing the copresentation of depression in patients with Alzheimer's disease is that depression in the demented patient is often hard to recognize. The pathoplastic effect, that is the impact of one pathology on the presentation of another, of the cognitive impairment on the presentation of the depressive illness as well as the inability of the impaired patient to comprehend or communicate symptoms accurately or consistently can be substantial. Therefore, the clinician cannot rely on the DSM-IIIR criteria which are more appropriate for cognitively-intact young adults but will have to focus instead on behavioral changes as well as the biological features of the disease.

Thus, the following would appear to be operational criteria for detecting depression in the presence of dementia.

- dysphoria, fatigue or anergia
- fitful sleep with frequent distressed wakenings
- poor appetite with loss of weight
- non-specific dysfunctional behaviour, e.g. agitation, aggression, pacing, yelling
- diurnal variation of dysfunctional behaviour ('sunrising')
- non-specific psychotic symptoms, commonly mood-congruent or paranoid

In our clinical experience the presence of three or more of these criteria for a period of more than two weeks should be grounds for a putative diagnosis of depression in cognitively-impaired patients.

Using these criteria, in a consecutive sample of 100 elderly patients admitted to the Geriatric Psychiatry inpatient unit, 41% were also depressed (Ancill, 1989b). More recently, we reviewed 291 consecutive admissions to our inpatient programme. Of these patients, using DSM-IIIR criteria which may have underestimated the 'true' incidence, 151 (52%) had a mood disorder and were depressed. There were 51 men and 100 women with a mean age of 76 (range 61–89). Of the 151 depressed patients, 93 (62%) were also demented, 36 men and 57 women with a mean age of 78 (range 61–85). Of the 93 patients with both depression and dementia, there were 35 patients (38%) whose depression predated the onset of their dementia and there were 58 (62%) whose depression came on after they became cognitively impaired.

Recognizing that we are looking at a selected population of patients referred for inpatient assessment or treatment, it is clear that depression, whether in the presence of a dementia or not, is common in the geriatric population. Of note in this study was that in the demented patients, depression was recognized in only 15% of cases by the referring physician and neuroleptics had been prescribed in 76 of the 91 (84%) patients with both dementia and depression, although psychotic features were present in less than 20% of those receiving antipsychotic drugs.

OUTCOME OF DEPRESSION IN THE ELDERLY

As was stated earlier, some authors have argued that therapeutic outcome in elderly depressed patients is poor. Murphy (1983) showed that in her sample, after one year, only 35% had recovered and a further 19% had recovered but relapsed. On the other hand, others have emphasized the treatability of depression in the elderly with recovery rates of between 58% and 86% (Baldwin and Jolley, 1986; Ancill, 1989b). More recent work by Kivela and Pahkala (1989) found an overall good clinical outcome in 50% of their sample and suggested that there may be two groups, one with better outcome. Associated with poorer outcome were such variables as presence of delusions, several life events in preceding year, not living alone (females), presence of agitation and poor social interaction. However these variables may reflect severity of depression and details of treatment protocols were not described, either for the acute phase or for maintenance. Clearly there is debate and confusion as to effective therapeutic strategies and outcome. Given this confusion, it is perhaps understandable why therapeutic nihilism impacts on this population given the diagnostic difficulties, a perception of poor outcome combined with increased risks of adverse events with standard biological treatments.

TREATMENT OF DEPRESSION IN THE ELDERLY

Generally speaking, the most likely treatment of depression in an elderly patient in Canada remains a tricyclic antidepressant, the most commonly used in this vulnerable age group being the tertiary amine tricyclic such as amitriptyline or doxepin (Ancill and Holliday, 1990). The major adverse events from these drugs impacting on the elderly include postural hypotension with the risk of falls and consequent fractures, and anticholinergic confusional states. For patients with the added burden of Alzheimer's disease, the use of anticholinergic medications must always be questioned and avoided whenever possible. Although the secondary amine tricyclics desipramine and nortriptyline have an improved side effects profile, they still retain significant toxicity and this has led many authorities to conclude that although the tricyclics are effective 'we clearly need better drugs' (Gerson et al., 1988).

Trazodone was the first non-tricyclic serotonergic antidepressant available in Canada. It is a post-synaptic 5HT agonist with marked sedative properties making it a good choice for agitated depression in an elderly patient who also has a sleep disturbance. It has a therapeutic blood range of 2000–6000 mmol/l and its side effects include hypotension and occasional acute confusional states. Early concerns about priapism have not been realized with wider use and in any event is not unknown with other antidepressants.

The recent introduction of presynaptic 5HT reuptake blockers (SRIs) has now substantially increased the choice of non-tricyclic agents available. Fluoxetine is stimulating and serotonergic side effects, such as nausea, diarrhoea and anxiety, are not uncommon in the elderly especially at the 20 mg dose. Initial dosing should perhaps be 5 mg. Its long-acting metabolite, norfluoxetine, can also be problematic although fluoxetine is clearly a 'safer' drug than the tricyclics. Fluvoxamine is less stimulating and has more favourable pharmacokinetics in the elderly than does fluoxetine. The initial dose in the elderly is 25 mg with maintenance around 100 mg given as a single dose at night. Side effects are serotonergic but generally milder than with fluoxetine. Sertraline is also a recently introduced SRI and is a mildly stimulating agent. In Canada, it is available as a 50 mg capsule and giving a reduced initial dose (25 mg) for the elderly is not easy. Therefore, initial side effects can be a problem in some older patients.

Buspirone, a non-benzodiazepine azapirone anxiolytic, is a serotonin partial agonist acting mainly at the $5HT_{1a}$ receptor. It can be effective in mixed anxiety–depression syndromes but it is not clear if buspirone is an antidepressant. Its side effects are milder than with the SRI group and initial dosage in the elderly is 5 mg. Maintenance dosage is between 20–40 mg per day. The most recent introduction of an antidepressant into Canada is that of moclobemide, a reversible MAO-A inhibitor with minimal tyramine reactivity. Therefore, dietary and drug precautions are not required. Given the likely widespread transmitter disturbances that are present in the depressed demented patient, there are theoretical reasons why an MAOI might be beneficial although more clinical data are required. Moclobemide has a good side effect profile in the elderly. The dose in the elderly is 150 mg twice a day, immediately after food.

Electroconvulsive therapy (ECT) remains an effective treatment for severe depression in the elderly whether they have a dementia or not. While 'pseudodementia' remains a controversial term (McAllister, 1983), some authors have demonstrated that effective treatment of an affective disorder can result either in full cognitive recovery (Rabins et al., 1984) or, more often, with some improvement in Mini-Mental State score in patients with both depression and dementia after resolution of the depressive syndrome (Ancill, 1989b). ECT has been shown to be beneficial in elderly patients presenting with both depression and dementia (Ancill, 1989b; Liang et al., 1988) and is indicated for depressed patients in the following situations.

- chemotherapy not effective
- chemotherapy not tolerated
- life threatened by refusing to eat or drink
- previous good response to ECT
- physical frailty where chemotherapy would be problematic
- acutely suicidal
- systematized delusions

ECT may also be effective in demented patients with severe dysfunctional behaviour, such as prolonged screaming, where other treatable conditions have been excluded and even where the depressive features are 'soft' or unclear (Carlyle et al., 1991).

Ideally, when acute treatment has resulted in a good clinical response, maintenance therapy will be required. How long this should go on for is unclear, especially if there is an organic basis for the mood disorder. However, for unipolar depressions, continuing with the antidepressant for at least six months after maximal resolution of symptoms is a reasonable strategy with a subsequent therapeutic trial of gradual reduction. Full acute phase dosage may need to be reinstated if relapse occurs. For bipolar patients, or those who cannot tolerate longer-term antidepressant therapy, lithium may be useful. Blood levels should probably be less than that for adults, around 0.2–0.5 mEq/l, and care should be taken to review thyroid and renal function regularly. Currently, there is insufficient information to make recommendations about other 'mood stabilizers' in the elderly such as carbamazepine or valproate although they have been used when lithium is either not effective or not tolerated.

Where ECT has been used in the acute phase, it may be necessary to consider its use for maintenance. In our programme we have a small number of demented patients whose depression resolves with ECT but who then relapse without continuing the ECT. Usually we are able slowly to increase the interval between treatments to monthly with the patient being treated as a day patient provided there is a care-giver who can ensure nil by mouth prior to the treatment. It is unfortunate that few centres offer ECT to elderly depressed patients and even fewer have maintenance ECT programmes.

In the study referred to earlier involving 151 depressed geriatric patients, 58 were depressed but were not demented (DND), 35 were depressed prior to the onset of the cognitive impairment (DBD) and 58 became depressed after the onset of the dementing disorder (DAD). Patients were treated using optimized protocols whereby the 'best choice' treatment was decided clinically for each patient. If this treatment failed or was not tolerated then the next indicated therapy was initiated. ECT was included in these protocols. Outcome was evaluated by an independent review of the patients' charts and was based on a Clinician's Global Impression (CGI).

Of the DND group, 52 patients (90%) improved and at six months follow-up only six (11.5%) had relapsed. In the DBD group where dementia postdated the onset of the mood disorder, 28 patients (80%) improved with four relapses (14%) over the next six months. In the DAD group where the dementia predated the depressive illness, 45 patients (77.5%) improved with acute therapy and seven patients (15.5%) relapsed over the next six months. These differences do not reach statistical difference but there is a trend for a marginal reduction of response rates and a marginal increase of relapse rates when depression copresents with dementia. However, the response rates remain generally high and relapse rates, at least over six months, are low overall.

CONCLUSIONS

The copresentation of depression in dementia is being increasingly recognized. The actual pathological relationship between the two syndromes is complex and multifactorial. The features of depression may well be altered by the presence of the cognitive impairment, but the diagnosis can still be made. There are a variety of effective and well-tolerated treatments available, including ECT. However, recent pharmaceutical advances have broadened the range of options for the clinician. The therapeutic nihilism of 'dementism' is perhaps the most significant problem the patient faces yet there is a substantial body of evidence demonstrating that the acute response of depression in the elderly, even in the presence of dementia, is high and longer-term prognosis is by no means hopeless. What confounds the situation is concern about effective treatments. Clinical data in this particular population are sparse yet there is an increasing awareness that depression in demented patients responds to acute treatment with improvement in affective symptoms and often in cognition as well. Where dysfunctional behaviour is the presenting problem, depression is one of the major underlying causes and the behaviour will improve as the depression resolves. This approach is preferable to the traditional intervention of 'behaviour modification' which does little to deal with underlying causative pathologies. There are legitimate concerns about the side effects of biological treatments. Because of age-related and disease-related pharmacokinetic and pharmacodynamic changes, chemotherapy is more likely to cause emergent adverse reactions. Antidepressant medications should be chosen primarily on their side effects profile and tailored for an individual patient. There is no one 'drug of choice' although there are many that should be avoided if possible. Serotonergic agents are better tolerated on balance than are the tricyclics although there may be some demented depressed patients with a primary noradrenergic pathology who might not be expected to respond to serotonergic antidepressants. ECT is a valuable treatment that should not be denied to patients for whom it is indicated both in the acute as well as maintenance phases.

Further work is clearly needed in this confounding and confusing area of geriatric psychiatry. Depression in patients with Alzheimer's disease and other neurodegenerative dementing disorders is diagnosable and treatable but only if time and care are taken to examine the mental state, elicit the features that are diagnostic and to optimize treatment.

REFERENCES

Agbayewa, M.O. (1986). Earlier psychiatric morbidity in patients with Alzheimer's disease. *J. Am. Geriatr. Soc.*, **34**, 561–564.

Ancill, R.J. (1989a). Dysfunctional behaviour in Alzheimer's disease. *Med. N. Am.*, **37**, 6662–6665.

Ancill, R.J. (1989b). Cognitive-affective disorders: the copresentation of depression and dementia in the elderly. *Psychiatr. J. Uni. Ottawa*, **14**, 370–371.

Ancill, R.J. and Holliday, S.G. (1990). Treatment of depression in the elderly: a Canadian view. *Prog. Neuropsychopharmacol. Biol. Psychiatry*, **14**, 655–661.

Ancill, R.J., Embury, G.D., MacEwan, G.W. and Kennedy, J.S. (1988). The use and misuse of psychotropic prescribing for elderly psychiatric patients. *Can. J. Psychiatry*, **33**, 585–589.

Baldwin, R.C. and Jolley, D.J. (1986). The prognosis of depression in old age. *Br. J. Psychiatry*, **149**, 574–583.

Carlyle, W., Killick, L. and Ancill, R.J. (1991). ECT: an effective treatment in the screaming demented patient. *J. Am. Geriatr. Soc.*, **39**, 637–639.

Cummings, J.L. (1992). Depression and Parkinson's disease: a review. *Am. J. Psychiatry*, **149**, 443–454.

Emory, V.O. and Oxman, T.E. (1992). Update on the dementia spectrum of depression. *Am. J. Psychiatry*, **149**, 305–317.

Gerson, S.C., Plotkin, D.A. and Jarvik, L.F. (1988). Antidepressant drug studies 1964–85: empirical evidence for aging patients. *J. Clin. Pharmacol.*, **8**, 311–322.

Kivela, S.-L. and Pahkala, K. (1989). The prognosis of depression in old age. *Int. J. Geriatr. Psychiatry*, **1**, 119–134.

Koenig, H.G., Goli, V., Shelp, F., Kudler, H.S., Cohen, H.J. and Blazer, D.G. (1992). Major depression in hospitalized medically ill older men: documentation, management and outcome. *Int. J. Geriatr. Psychiatry*, **7**, 25–34.

Lazarus, L.W., Newton, N., Cohler, B., Lesser, J. and Schweon, C. (1987). Frequency and presentation of depressive symptoms in patients with primary degenerative dementia. *Am. J. Psychiatry*, **144**, 41–45.

Liang, R.A., Lam, R.W. and Ancill, R.J. (1988). ECT in the treatment of mixed depression and dementia. *Br. J. Psychiatry*, **152**, 281–284.

Liston, E.H. (1978). Diagnostic delay in presenile dementia. *J. Clin. Psychiatry*, **39**, 599–603.

McAllister, T.W. (1983). Overview: pseudodementia. *Am. J. Psychiatry*, **140**, 528–533.

Murphy, E. (1983). The prognosis of depression in old age. *Br. J. Psychiatry*, **142**, 111–119.

Rabins, P.V., Merchant, A. and Nestadt, G. (1984). Criteria for diagnosing reversible dementia caused by depression. *Br. J. Psychiatry*, **144**, 488–492.

Reifler, B.V. (1986). Mixed cognitive–affective disturbances in the elderly: a new classification. *J. Clin. Psychiatry*, **47**, 354–356.

Wells, C.E. (1979). Pseudodementia. *Am. J. Psychiatry*, **136**, 895–900.

Zweig, R.M., Ross, C.A. and Hedreen, J.C. *et al.* (1993). The neuropathology of aminergic nuclei in Alzheimer's disease. *Ann. Neurol.*, in press.

9

Alzheimer's Disease: Cognitive Assessment and Therapeutic Strategies in France

J.-F. DÉMONET, P. CELSIS AND B. GUIRAUD-CHAUMEIL

INSERM U 230 and Service de Neurologie, Hopital Purpan, Toulouse, France

INTRODUCTION

Neurologists and neuropsychologists may hesitate when facing the choice of appropriate cognitive tools for the assessment of demented patients' performance. Indeed, at a first glance, a large number of neuropsychological tests seem available. However, very few of them appear to be suitable for specific purposes, such as (a) early diagnosis of dementia, (b) specific diagnosis of dementia of Alzheimer type (DAT), or (c) follow-up studies. The number of suitable tests becomes even smaller when one considers the methodological issues of therapeutic trials in dementias of Alzheimer type. Nevertheless, many of these trials have been undertaken, using batteries of inadequate tests, leading to prolonged sessions of cognitive testing which mean increasing discomfort and unreliable cognitive performance for both patients and examiners.

It might be that such methodological errors precluded the identification of small cognitive effects of some compounds which have been tested in demented patients. In fact, the absence of precise guidelines for cognitive testing probably reflects the poor level of our knowledge of all aspects of dementias, from their neurobiological to their cognitive dimensions.

However, research is very active in this field and advances in various domains will probably allow us to solve these methodological problems. In this chapter, only some of the recent relevant issues as well as their implications for the methodology of therapeutic trials will be addressed.

EARLY DIAGNOSIS

One of the most important issues in this topic is to ensure an *accurate diagnosis of DAT during the early stages* of the disease because the potential effects of drugs would be more important at these stages than at later stages. This issue is connected with the problem of inclusion criteria and the constitution of homogeneous samples of patients in multi-centre trials. According to recent studies (Joachim and Selkoe, 1992), stratification of patient samples should be made according to some important clinical features such as the presence of a familial history of dementia, early versus late onset of dementia, and the existence of neurological abnormalities, particularly myoclonias or abnormalities of tone.

With regard to the diagnosis of cognitive impairment, the diagnostic criteria identified in formal check-lists such as the DSM-IIIR or the NINCDS–ADRDA criteria are, by far, neither sensitive nor specific enough to achieve an early diagnosis, and cognitive tests are always necessary to provide objective evidence supporting clinical impressions.

Some authors (Eslinger *et al.*, 1975; Storandt *et al.*, 1984) identified sets of neuropsychological tests which would allow an early diagnosis of DAT (Table 1). These tests explore memory and attention processes for both verbal and non-verbal stimuli. This is also consistent with a more recent study (Welsh *et al.*, 1991) which emphasized the sensitivity of the delayed recall of a list of 10 words. However, such tasks are also highly sensitive to changes observed in normal ageing (Claman and Sluss-Radebaugh, 1991). This emphasizes the crucial importance in large-scale studies of investigating cognitive and behavioural changes in ageing populations. These studies suggest that cognitive performance in the simple tests largely used in screening procedures may be affected by factors such as age and level of education.

Figure 1 displays a result from one of our studies on cognitive performance in normal subjects (Démonet *et al.*, 1990) and demonstrates the influence of level of education and age on one of the most important items of the Folstein

Table 1. Early diagnosis of dementias of Alzheimer type.

Eslinger et al. (1975)	Storandt et al. (1984)
Orientation[a]	Mental control[a]
Digit span[a]	Logical memory[a]
Logical memory[a]	Verbal fluency
Paired word learning[a]	Trail making test (A)[c]
Visual retention test[b]	
Verbal fluency	
Face recognition test[b]	
Line orientation test[b]	

[a]Wechsler Memory Scale.
[b]From Benton (1974), Benton and Van Allen (1973), and Benton *et al.* (1975).
[c]From Reitan (1958).

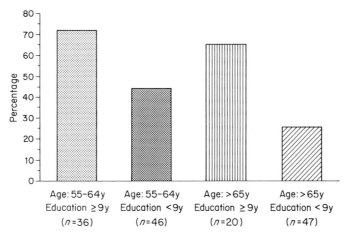

Figure 1.   Percentage of normal subjects achieving five serial subtractions of 7 from 100, according to age and level of education.

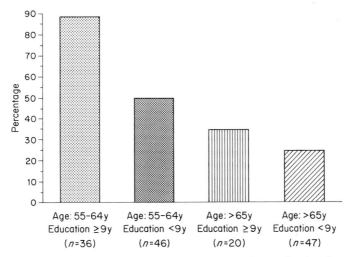

Figure 2.   Percentage of normal subjects copying correctly a cube drawing, according to age and level of education.

MMS: the five steps of serial subtractions of 7 from 100. Whereas age does not seem to influence such performance very much, the effect of educational level is important in these normal subjects.

Another example is the ability to copy a cube with an adequate rendering of the third dimension. This test is very frequently used in clinical practice and is an item of the Alzheimer's Disease Assessment Scale designed by Rosen and colleagues. As displayed in Fig. 2, both age and educational level seem to affect performance on this test. These data have been acquired in a sample of 149 subjects but we are taking part in a very much larger survey called PAQUID conducted by Dartigues and colleagues from the INSERM (Bordeaux) and their first results on this test seem to confirm our previous ones.

These results demonstrated that basic epidemiological factors may exert a profound influence on tests used in the first stages of trial protocols and the influence of these factors should be considered when inclusion criteria are discussed. This concerns particularly scores on Folstein MMS which are sensitive to educational factors. Although still controversial, the existence of an influence of these factors on dementia manifestations has been recently emphasized by some authors (Stern *et al.*, 1992).

ASSESSMENT OF CHANGES IN COGNITIVE FUNCTIONS

The cornerstone of therapeutic trials consists of one (or several) neuropsychological tests selected to assess cognitive impairments at the beginning of the study and further changes in patients' cognitive status. The choice of the tests depends on the objectives of the study. Most studies aim to assess the effects of a compound on cognition in general and global cognitive scales are used for this purpose. Alternatively, drug effects may be investigated in a particular cognitive domain of general memory processes and these studies resort to specific cognitive tests.

Many different global cognitive scales have been used such as the Blessed Scale, the Dementia Rating Scale, or the Alzheimer's Disease Assessment Scale. The latter is becoming more widely used in therapeutic trials following the recommendation of the American FDA. The use of such global scales gives rise to many methodological problems. First of all, their sensitivity to possible cognitive changes may vary from one stage of severity to another and this emphasizes the importance of the homogeneity of patient samples in a study. Moreover, according to Salmon and colleagues (1990), the ability of these scales to evaluate longitudinal changes in patients seems disputable and is still to be confirmed.

Another pitfall of large-scale, cooperative, multi-centre trials consists of the cross-cultural and cross-linguistic problems which do not allow the use of simple translations of scales into another language. Our group participated in the translation and the adaptation of the Alzheimer's Disease Scale. The items of this memory sub-test have been selected according to language criteria such as lexical frequency, picturability, phonological structure and semantic relationships, all of which are of course peculiar to French language (Dérouesné *et al.*, 1992, unpublished). Control data must now be acquired with this version in a population of normal ageing, French-speaking subjects.

HETEROGENEITY OF THE DEMENTIAS OF ALZHEIMER TYPE

The major disadvantage of the use of global cognitive scales is related to the heterogeneity of DAT. Heterogeneity is probably the most important issue in methodology of therapeutic trials. Heterogeneity is now well recognized (Boller *et al.*, 1992) and appears to be multi-dimensional with genetic, clinical, metabolic and neuropsychological aspects.

From a neuropsychological point of view, the heterogeneity of the primary degenerative dementias may, to some extent, reflect some cognitive heterogeneities which seem to exist in a normal, ageing population, and possibly different cognitive styles, as suggested by a recent study of Valdois and colleagues (1990).

Our group designed a correlational approach to different aspects of the heterogeneity by combining neuropsychological, EEG and single photon emission tomography (SPECT) studies of a series of DAT patients which now involves about a hundred subjects. All these patients were thought to present a probable DAT according to the DSM-IIIR and the NINCDS–ADRDA criteria. However, they demonstrated massive heterogeneity.

In the first 20 patients included in this series, significant correlations were observed between cognitive, EEG and regional cerebral blood flow (rCBF) scores of inter-hemispheric asymmetry (Celsis *et al.*, 1990), suggesting a good concordance between cognitive measurements and biological evidence of left/right asymmetry of brain dysfunction. These scores are derived from comparisons between data observed in these patients and a control group of ageing, normal subjects who are also currently involved in a follow-up study. A cognitive asymmetry score has been designed from various standardized tests reflecting dysfunctions of either left or right cerebral hemispheres.

These results have been further confirmed in a larger series using SPECT (Celsis *et al.*, 1991) or positron emission tomography (PET) (Haxby *et al.*, 1988). More importantly, in this group of 91 patients (Fig. 3), SPECT data demonstrated that only 35 patients (38% of this group) did not present significant inter-regional differences in rCBF deficits, suggesting diffuse and homogeneous changes in the brain. Significant regional preponderances of cerebral blood flow decrease were found in 56 patients (61%), with a large subgroup of 31 asymmetric cases having left hemispheric deficits. Moreover, among the 27 patients presenting no lateral asymmetry (on the medial line of Fig. 3), 16 cases presented a hypoperfusion significantly more marked in the posterior parietal regions than in the frontal regions. A preponderance of rCBF deficits in the frontal regions was observed in eight patients.

The so-called 'deep' subgroup consists of cases in which rCBF values were significantly lower in the subcortical regions than in the cortical regions. In this subgroup (Table 2), most patients were women, the age-at-onset and the

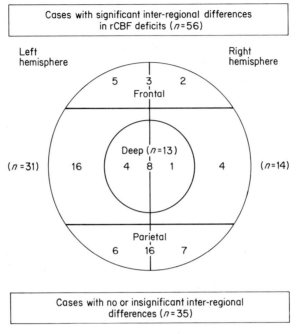

Figure 3. Topographical subgroups of 91 DAT patients according to the regional preponderance of rCBF deficit measured with single photon emission tomography.

Folstein MMS score were higher and deficits of symbolic functions (such as language and praxis) were less marked than in other subgroups of patients. In fact, these 'deep' patients presented predominantly memory disorders.

As far as therapeutic trials are concerned, these data strongly suggest that (a) the usual criteria used for inclusion may select not only Alzheimer's

Table 2.   Clinical and neuropsychological data in a group of 91 DAT patients (from Celsis *et al.*, 1991).[a]

Regional preponderance of rCBF deficits	Posterior (n=29)	Anterior (n=10)	Deep (n=13)	Borderline (n=19)	
Sex ratio (M/F)	17/12	3/7	2/11	5/14	
Age at onset	63	67.5	71.3	61.4	$p<0.05$
Folstein MMS	13.8	13.6	16.5	22.0	$p<0.01$
Symbolic deficit	5.6	5.4	3.8	3.6	$p<0.01$
Memory deficit	5.5	5.0	4.6	4.6	n.s.

[a]Patients not included in this table presented either normal pattern or focal deficits.

disease cases but also other primary degenerative dementias such as frontal lobe dementias, (b) patients pertaining to these different subgroups should not be included in the same pool and (c) some subgroups, for instance the 'deep' subgroup with a predominance of memory disorders might be particular targets for the assessment of the effects of specific compounds such as cholinomimetics.

PET may also be used in normal subjects to differentiate the neural correlates of different cognitive functions. We recently studied (Démonet et al., 1992) brain areas significantly activated in normal subjects during two different language tasks, a lexicosemantic and a phonological task which explore, respectively, two modes of verbal memory. Lexicosemantic processes related to long-term semantic memory activate various cortical areas in the frontal, temporal and parietal association cortex in the left and even in the right hemisphere. The phonological task elicits processes of short-term working memory and their brain correlates are less widely distributed, involving only the left inferior parietal region. All these foci of activation are association cortex areas which are frequently damaged in Alzheimer's disease. Different patterns of memory impairment have been described in DAT patients, with more or less pronounced deficits of short-term memory or long-term memory (Van der Linden et al., 1991). These different patterns may correspond to differences in the topography of lesions which would predominate either in juxta-sylvian areas or in other association neocortical areas.

In summary, specific cognitive impairments characterized in subgroups of DAT patients in their multiple facets (genetics, neuropsychology, brain mapping, etc.), should ideally be assessed by specific neuropsychological tasks which would be standardized in normal controls according to language and cultural peculiarities. Only such an approach will allow us to detect relevant changes in cognitive performance between the different groups particularly in a drug study protocol.

CONCLUSION

Many of the new concepts provided by different domains of research into Alzheimer's disease should be considered in the design of therapeutic trials. Most issues which have been addressed in this chapter reflect our own experience; however, there is an increasing endeavour to obtain a consensus about the methodology of therapeutic trials among French teams undertaking clinical research on DAT. The ideal conditions for studies of cognitive changes which have been mentioned require large and difficult research programmes and pharmaceutical companies should certainly participate in and support even preliminary steps such as normalization and validation of new cognitive tools suitable for therapeutic trials.

REFERENCES

Benton, A.L. (1974). *The Revised Visual Retention Test, 4th edn.* Psychological Corporation, New York.

Benton, A.L. and Van Allen, M.W. (1973). *Test of Facial Recognition Manual.* Neurosensory Center Publication No. 287, University of Iowa.

Benton, A.L., Hannay, H.J. and Varnay, N.R. (1975). Visual perception of line direction in patients with unilateral brain disease. *Neurology*, **25**, 907–910.

Boller, F., Forette, F., Khachaturian, Z., Poncet, M. and Christen, Y. (1992). *Heterogeneity of Alzheimer's Disease.* Springer-Verlag, Berlin, Heidelberg.

Celsis, P., Agniel, A., Puel, M., Le Tinnier, A., Viallard, G., Démonet, J.-F., Rascol, A. and Marc-Vergnes, J-P. (1990). Lateral asymmetries in primary degenerative dementia of the Alzheimer type. A correlative study of cognitive, haemodynamic and EEG data, in relation with severity, age of onset and sex. *Cortex*, **26**, 585–596.

Celsis, P., Agniel, A., Puel, M., Démonet, J.-F., Rascol, A. and Marc-Vergnes, J.-P. (1991). Hemodynamic subtypes of dementia of the Alzheimer type: clinical and neuropsychological characteristics. In: Rapoport, S.R., Petit, H., Leys, D. and Christen, Y. (Eds), *Imaging, Cerebral Topography and Alzheimer's Disease*, Springer-Verlag, Berlin, pp. 145–157.

Claman, D.L. and Sluss-Radebaugh, T. (1991). Neuropsychological assessment in clinical trials of Alzheimer's disease. *Alzheimer's Dis. Assoc. Disord.*, **5** (Suppl. 1), S49–S56.

Démonet, J.-F., Doyon, B., Ousset, P.-J., Puel, M., Mahagne, M.-H., Cardebat, D., Duchein, C., Viala, M.-F., Agniel, A., Vellas, B. and Rascol, A. (1990). Evaluation des fonctions cognitives dans les démences: étalonnage d'une échelle modulaire et hiérarchisée. *Rev. Neurol.*, **146**, 490–501.

Démonet, J.-F., Chollet, F., Ramsay, S., Cardebat, D., Nespoulous, J.-L., Wise, R., Rascol, A. and Frackowiak, R. (1992). The anatomy of phonological and semantic processing in normal subjects. *Brain*, **115**, 1753–1768.

Eslinger, P.J., Damasio, A.R., Benton, A.L. and Van Allen, M. (1975). Neuropsychologic detection of abnormal decline in older persons. *J. Am. Med. Assoc.*, **5**, 670–674.

Haxby, J.V., Grady, C.L., Koss, E., Horwitz, B., Schapiro, M., Friedland, R.P. and Rapoport, S.R. (1988). Heterogeneous anterior–posterior metabolic patterns in dementia of the Alzheimer type. *Neurology*, **38**, 1853–1863.

Joachim, C.L. and Selkoe, D.J. (1992). The seminal role of beta-amyloid in the pathogenesis of Alzheimer disease. *Alzheimer Dis. Relat. Disord.*, **6**, 7–34.

Reitan, R.M. (1958). Validity of the trial making test as an indicator of organic brain damage. *Percept. Mot. Skills*, **8**, 271–276.

Salmon, D.P., Thal, L.J., Butters, N. and Heindel, W.C. (1990). Longitudinal evaluation of dementia of the Alzheimer type: a comparison of 3 standardized mental status examination. *Neurology*, **40**, 1225–1230.

Stern, Y., Andrews, H., Pittman, J., Sano, M., Tatemichi, T., Lantiga, R. and Mayeaux, R. (1992). Diagnosis of dementia in a heterogeneous population. Development of a neuropsychological paradigm-based diagnosis of dementia and quantified correction for the effects of education. *Arch. Neurol.*, **49**, 453–460.

Storandt, M., Botwinick, J., Danziger, W.L., Berg, L. and Hughes, C.P. (1984). Psychometric differentiation of mild senile dementia of the Alzheimer type. *Arch. Neurol.*, **41**, 497–499.

Valdois, S., Joanette, Y., Possant, Y., Ska, B. and Dehaut, F. (1990). Heterogeneity in the cognitive profile of normal elderly. *J. Clin. Exp. Neuropsychol.*, **12**, 587–596.

Van der Linden, M., Ansay, C., Calicis, F., Jacquemin, A., Schils, J.-P., Seron, X. and Wyns, C. (1991). Prise en charge des déficits cognitifs dans la démence d'Alzheimer. In: Habib, M., Joanette, Y. and Puel, M. (Eds), *Dédemces et Syndromes Démentiels: Approche Neuropsychologique.* Masson, Paris, pp. 253–262.

Welsh, K.A., Butters, N., Hughes, J., Mohs, R. and Heyman, A. (1991). Detection of abnormal memory decline in mild cases of Alzheimer's disease using CERAD neuropsychological measures. *Arch. Neurol.*, **48**, 278–281.

The Management of Alzheimer's Disease
Edited by Gordon K. Wilcock
©1993 Wrightson Biomedical Publishing Ltd

10

Alzheimer's Disease: Caring and Pharmacological Treatment Strategies in Sweden

BENGT WINBLAD, HEDDA AGUERO TORRES, KJERSTIN ERICSSON,
LAURA FRATIGLIONI AND AGNETA NORDBERG

*Stockholm Gerontology Research Center and Department of Geriatric Medicine,
Karolinska Institute, Stockholm, Sweden*

INTRODUCTION

The number of elderly people, particularly those aged over 75 years, constitutes an increasing proportion of the total population in most developed countries. The particular disabilities of this group become more and more relevant for researchers and to those who provide health care and social services. Dementia is a frequent condition among the elderly, and the most devastating among the age-related diseases of the brain. For these reasons, dementia is important not only for the effects on the individual patients and on their families, but also on society.

The management of demented patients is complex. Behavioural and cognitive deficits always require care, but only some symptoms are responsive to psychopharmacological treatment. For this reason good care has become of great importance in the treatment of these patients as well as pharmacological intervention. While clinical trials are the studies that we need in order to test the efficacy of a new drug, epidemiological studies supply data for planning general health services. Since the care needs of demented elderly are associated with the level of cognitive impairment (Aronson *et al.*, 1992), prevalence of the disease, specific for degree of severity, can be used for the judgement of the quantitative and qualitative aspects of the care of the demented subjects in the community and in institutions.

CARE OF THE ELDERLY IN SWEDEN

Care of the elderly is one of the cornerstones of the Swedish welfare society. The modern era of care for the elderly arose during the 1950s. In this period many institutions for the elderly were built, but because of economic and humanitarian reasons this policy was questioned during the late 1960s. In the early 1970s, a new era of home-based care for elderly people started. After that, during the 1980s, because more dependent elderly received help in their own homes, there was a decline in the demand for traditional institutional care with increased demands for intermediate forms of institutional housing. Now, at the beginning of 1990s, the strategic task is to try to develop the existing care system through modernization and rationalization, with less costly care alternatives and, at the same time, develop support for the cooperation with the informal care system (Johansson and Thorslund, 1991).

Like the cognitively intact elderly, patients with dementia disorders are looked after in either home care or in local nursing homes. However, to improve dementia care, some alternatives in the organization of the medical systems have been proposed. These include assessment units, homes and home care with relief for the care-giver, homes with day and/or night care, homes with relief care, sheltered housing, sheltered wards in old people's homes, nursing homes and special units for patients with extremely disturbed behaviour. However, at present these facilities are too few in number and the rate of building is far too slow to keep up with the increasing number of patients.

CARING FOR A DEMENTED PERSON

The interaction between the care-giver, the patient and the family is of extreme importance when caring for Alzheimer's disease patients. It is the central part of the philosophy of care. To be sensitive and have empathy helps the care-giver in understanding patients' altered needs, due to the progression of the disease (Sandman, 1990). In the caring situation the care-givers can experience a conflict between the care they would like to provide and the care they actually give (Hallberg, 1990). Therefore the care-givers have an acute need for professional counselling and support. Counselling at the time of diagnosis should be comprehensive with planned support provided regularly even during the progression of the disease. Family members caring for parents or spouses with Alzheimer's disease play a pivotal role in long-term care. Their attitude, knowledge and utilization of community resources can determine the quality of care that Alzheimer's patients receive. Mild cases of Alzheimer's disease have the greatest chance of maintaining their social and mental function when enabled to maintain their familiar home surroundings. Therefore home care seems to be the principal aim for the majority of the demented. In this case, they need the availability of day-care centres where they can be active together with others in a psychosocially and physically stimulating environment. This will offer them the possibility of utilizing their existing skills. At the same time, the day-care centre will give support and relief to their relatives.

In a recent study performed in a district of Stockholm (Grafström *et al.*, 1992), all the relatives of the subjects with cognitive impairment, living at home, were compared with relatives of elderly, mentally healthy persons, living at home in the same district. The relatives of the demented subjects had more frequent subjective feelings of burden and greater use of psychotropic drugs. Spouses were the most stressed. However, they used medical facilities and somatic drugs to the same extent.

It has been stressed that availability of family support is a critical factor in predicting placement of chronically ill/disabled elderly, although there are some other characteristics observed in elderly subjects which are involved in the institutionalization process such as forgetfulness and confusion (Berg *et al.*, 1988), communication difficulties (Booth, 1986; Athlin and Norberg, 1987; Stoller and Pugliesi, 1988) and dependency in activities of daily living (Cherry and Rafkin, 1988).

Nursing home care should provide programmes specifically to avoid the understimulation which is frequently encountered particularly in demented elderly patients living in institutions. One way to ameliorate understimulation is to stimulate social interaction with other people. By using the patient group as a resource, we could introduce a change in attitude of the staff towards the patient, who is usually willing and capable of doing more than the staff generally believe. There must always be a balance between the patient's self-care capability and the help provided by the care-giver. We must be careful not to induce what has been labelled 'learned helplessness' and thus be at risk of progressing, through a series of events known as 'the social breakdown syndrome', to a completely dependent and inactive state (Kuypers and Bengtson, 1973).

PREVALENCE OF DEMENTIA AND CARE OF THE PATIENTS IN A SWEDISH URBAN POPULATION

In 1987 we startd a longitudinal study in Stockholm concerning ageing in general and related medical, psychological, and social problems in a population over 74 years old (the Kungsholmen project). This project was initiated also as a response to the need for basic epidemiological and health service information about psychiatric morbidity in Stockholm (Fratiglioni *et al.*, 1992a).

The observed prevalence of dementia was 7.2 and 16.3 per 100 men in the age groups 75–84 and over 84 years, respectively; and 7.6 and 25.9 per 100 women in the two age groups, respectively (Fratiglioni *et al.*, 1991). DSM-IIIR criteria for dementia were followed (Fratiglioni *et al.*, 1992b). The dementia staging was made following the Clinical Dementia Rating scale (CDR) (Hughes *et al.*, 1982) with some modifications (Forsell *et al.*, 1992). The prevalence of questionable, mild, moderate and severe dementia was equal to 1.0, 3.1, 5.5, and 2.3 per 100, respectively, with higher figures for the moderate–severe forms in advanced ages.

A review of the literature about institutionalization of demented elderly showed that the overwhelming majority of dementia cases are cared for in the community, even the severely demented (Preston, 1986). In contrast, data from the Kungsholmen project demonstrate that as many demented people lived in institutions as at home. When the degree of the disease severity is considered, most of the subjects with questionable–mild dementia (84%) live in their own homes, while most of the moderate–severe cases (77%) are institutionalized (Table 1).

Of the demented elderly who were living at home, 69% were living alone. Of those who were living with someone else, 83% were living with her or his partner, 10% with the children and 7% with another relative (Table 2).

Table 1. Distribution of demented elderly, by living place and severity of disease (CDR), number of cases (*n*) and proportion (%).

	Home		Home for elderly		Nursing home and long-stay ward	
CDR	*n*	*(%)*	*n*	*(%)*	*n*	*(%)*
Questionable	21	(20.8)	1	(5.6)	1	(1.0)
Mild	48	(47.5)	6	(33.3)	6	(5.7)
Moderate	28	(27.7)	11	(61.1)	60	(57.1)
Severe	4	(4.0)	0	(0.0)	38	(36.2)
Total	101	(100.0)	18	(100.0)	105	(100.0)

Table 2. Distribution of the elderly people living at home in the Kungsholmen population: demented, non-demented and total population and their living conditions, number of cases (*n*) and proportion (%).

	Alone		With someone else		Total	
	n	*(%)*	*n*	*(%)*	*n*	*(%)*
All population	1093	(70)	464	(30)	1557	(100)
Non-demented	1026	(70)	434	(30)	1460	(100)
Demented						
Questionable–mild	45	(66)	23	(34)	68	(100)
Moderate–severe	22	(76)	7	(24)	29	(100)

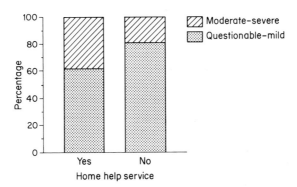

Figure 1. Proportion of demented elderly persons living at home, by degree of severity and presence of home help service.

Every Swedish municipality can provide a home help service to assist the elderly, i.e. cleaning, cooking, laundry, personal care and to some extent medical care (e.g. injections). Assistance may also be provided in the evenings and at night. In our population we found that 52% of the demented elderly who were living at home did not have such assistance. Among them, 19% had a moderate–severe form of dementia (Fig. 1).

Since 1969 in Sweden, the number of working hours of home help given to the elderly and to those with handicaps has steadily increased. In that year, around 35 million hours of home help were given, compared with 94 million hours in 1988. There is no information about the average number of hours per week worked by part-time employees. The Kungsholmen project's data show that 72% of the demented elderly who were living at home and had home held service had between 1 and 10 hours per week, 21% between 11 and 20 hours per week, and only 7% had more than 21 hours per week. Of those who had moderate–severe dementia, only 50% had more than 10 hours per week of home help service.

PHARMACOLOGICAL TREATMENT

Pharmacological treatment strategies in Alzheimer's disease are directed toward either cognitive or non-cognitive symptoms. Considerable progress has been made concerning non-cognitive behavioural and psychiatric symptoms. However, in spite of great efforts, no significant improvements in the cognitive impairment have been observed in clinical trials on Alzheimer's disease. Many pharmacological treatment strategies have been tried in dementia disorders: vasodilators, anticoagulants, psychostimulants, nootropics, cholinergic, monoaminergic and GABA-ergic drugs, neuropeptides, calcium channel blockers and copper- and aluminium-chelators.

At present, in our clinic, three major therapeutic approaches for the treatment of the cognitive symptoms of Alzheimer's disease are being studied:

- improvement of neurotransmission with THA (tetrahydroaminoacridine),
- stimulation of neuronal growth with NGF (nerve growth factor), and
- interruption of amyloid production/gene therapy.

THA treatment in Alzheimer's disease

In a recent study (Nordberg et al., 1993), we treated three patients with Alzheimer's disease, a 68 year-old woman with mild dementia and two men (64 and 72 years of age) with moderate dementia with oral THA, 80 mg daily, for several months. The patients were investigated using positron emission tomography (PET) prior to, and after three weeks and three months of treatment. In the PET studies we used [^{18}F]-fluorodeoxyglucose (^{18}F-FDG) (tracer for glucose metabolism), ^{11}C-butanol (cerebral blood flow) and (S)(–)- and (R)(+)-[N-^{11}C-methyl]-nicotine (nicotinic receptors, cholinergic neural activity).

THA treatment increased the uptake of ^{11}C-nicotine to the brain. A significantly reduced uptake between the two enantiomers (S)(–)- and (R)(+)^{11}C-nicotine was observed in the frontal and temporal cortices after THA treatment in all three patients. The kinetic analysis indicated increased binding of (S)(–)^{11}C-nicotine in brain compatible with restoration of nicotinic cholinergic receptors. The most pronounced effect was observed after three weeks and three months of treatment in the patient with mild dementia. An increase in cerebral glucose utilization was found in the 68 year-old patient with mild dementia but also slightly in the 64 year-old man with moderate dementia. THA administration did not affect cerebral blood flow. The PET data obtained after three weeks of THA treatment was paralleled by improvement in neuropsychological performance.

This PET study shows *in vivo* the induction of neurochemical effects in the brain by THA treatment in Alzheimer's disease patients. Intervention with THA in the early course of the disease might be necessary for a significant clinical improvement.

NGF treatment in Alzheimer's disease

The discovery by Levi-Montalcini (1964) of NFG has given us a valuable tool with which to study neuronal cell differentiation and growth.

Based on animal research suggesting that NGF can stimulate central cholinergic neurons, the known loss of cholinergic innervation in the cortex in Alzheimer's disease, and our experience of infusing NGF to support adrenal grafts in parkinsonian patients, we were able to perform NGF infusion into the brain of a patient with Alzheimer's disease (Olson et al., 1992). The case was a 69 year-old woman who had had symptoms of dementia for eight years. Intraventricular infusion of 6.6 mg NFG over three months resulted in a marked transient increase in uptake and binding of ^{11}C-nicotine in frontal and temporal cortex and a persistent increase in a cortical blood flow as measured by PET as well as progressive decrease of slow wave EEG activity. After one month of NGF, tests of verbal episodic memory had improved whereas other cognitive tests had not. No adverse effects could be ascribed to the NGF infusion.

The results of this case study indicate that NGF may counteract cholinergic deficits in Alzheimer's disease, and suggest that further trials of NGF infusion in Alzheimer's disease are warranted.

Amyloid in the pathogenesis of Alzheimer's disease

Whilst it was thought for many years that Alzheimer's disease was a heterogeneous disorder based on the clinical and neuropathological features of the disease, it was not until the techniques of molecular genetics were applied to this field that the question of heterogeneity was definitely proven. The identification by Hardy and colleagues (Goate et al., 1991) of a mutation in the amyloid precursor protein gene in some families was a valuable contribution to the field of Alzheimer's disease research. Although, the mutations at codon 717 in exon 17 of the ß-amyloid precursor protein (APP) gene in chromosome 21 have been shown in only a few families with early onset of Alzheimer's disease, their importance should not be underestimated. This mutation is the first known cause of the disease and confirms that amyloid deposition is a central event in the aetiology of the disorder.

We have recently (Mullan et al., 1992) identified on chromosome 21 a double mutation at codons 670 and 671 (APP 770 transcript) in exon 16 which co-segregates with the disease in two large (probably related) early-onset Alzheimer's disease families from Sweden. Two base pair transversions (G to T, A to C) from the normal sequence predict Lys to Asn and Met to Leu amino acid substitutions at codons 670 and 671 of APP transcript. This mutation occurs at the amino terminal of ß-amyloid and may be pathogenic because it occurs at or close to the endosomal/lysosomal cleavage site of the molecule. Thus, pathogenic mutations in APP frame the ß-amyloid sequence.

These findings have been largely responsible for the major refocusing of research activities into determining how ß-amyloid deposition results in the disease. Focusing on this aspect of the disease represents a promising avenue both for understanding the aetiology of the disorder as well as for the potential development of new therapeutic strategies aimed at delaying the onset and slowing the progression of the disease.

ACKNOWLEDGEMENTS

These studies were supported by grants from the Swedish Medical Research Council, the 'Gamla Tjänarinnor' Foundation, the 'Sveriges Kommunalanstaälldas Pensionskassa', Petrus and Augusta Hedlands Foundation, Loo and Hans Ostermans Foundation, Sigurd and Elsa Golje's Foundation.

REFERENCES

American Psychiatric Association (1987). *Diagnostic and Statistical Manual of Mental Disorders, 3rd edn, revised (DSM-III-R)*. American Psychiatric Association, Washington DC, pp. 97–163.

Aronson, M.K., Cox, D., Guastadisegni, P., Frazier, C., Sherlock, L., Grower, R., Barbera, A., Sternberg, M., Breed, J. and Koren, M.J. (1992). Dementia and nursing home: association with care needs. *J. Am. Geriatr. Soc.*, **40**, 27–33.

Athlin, E. and Norberg, A. (1987). Interaction between the severely demented patient and his caregiver during feeding. A theoretical model. *Scand. J. Caring. Sci.*, **1**, 117–123.

Berg, S., Branch, L.G., Doyle, A.E. and Sundström, G. (1988). Institutional and home-based long-term care alternatives: the 1965–1985 Swedish experience. *Gerontologist*, **28**, 825–829.

Booth, T. (1986). Institutional regimes and induced dependency in homes for the aged. *Gerontologist*, **26**, 418–423.

Cherry, D.L. and Rafkin, M.J. (1988). Adapting day care to the needs of adults with dementia. *Gerontologist*, **28**, 116–120.

Forsell, Y., Fratiglioni, L., Grut, M., Viitanen, M. and Winblad, B. (1992). Clinical staging of dementia in a population survey: comparison of DSM III-R and the Washington University Clinical Dementia Rating scale. *Acta Psychiatr. Scand.*, **86**, 49–54.

Fratiglioni, L., Grut, M., Forsell, Y., Grafström, M., Holmén, K., Eriksson, K., Viitanen, M., Blackman, L., Ahlbom, A. and Winblad, B. (1991). Prevalence of Alzheimer's disease and other dementias in an elderly urban population: relationship with age, sex and education. *Neurology*, **41**, 1886–1892.

Fratiglioni, L., Viitanen, M., Blackman, L., Sandman, P.O. and Winblad, B. (1992a). Occurrence of dementia in advanced age: the study design of the Kungsholmen project. *Neuroepidemiology*, **11** (Suppl. 1), 29–36.

Fratiglioni, L., Grut, M., Forsell, Y., Viitanen, M. and Winblad, B. (1992b). Clinical diagnosis of Alzheimer's disease and other dementias in a population survey. Agreement and causes of disagreement in applying DSM III-R criteria. *Arch. Neurol.*, **49**, 227–232.

Goate, A., Chartier-Harlin, M.C., Mullan, M., Brown, J., Crawford, F., Fidani, L., Giuffra, L., Haynes, A., Irving, N. and James, L. (1991). Segregation of a missense mutation in the amyloid precursor protein gene with familial Alzheimer's disease. *Nature*, **349**, 704–706.

Grafström, M., Fratiglioni, L., Sandman, P.O. and Winblad, B. (1992). Health and social consequences for relatives of demented and nondemented elderly. A population-based study. *J. Clin. Epidemiol.*, **45**, 861–870.

Hallberg, I.R. (1990). *Vocally Disruptive Behaviour in Severely Demented Patients in Relation to Institutional Care Provided.* Department of Advanced Nursing, Umeå University Medical Dissertations. New Series No. 261.

Hughes, C.P., Berg, L., Danzinger, W.L., Coben, L.A. and Martin, R.L. (1982). A new clinical scale for staging of dementia. *Br. J. Psychiatry*, **140**, 566–572.

Johansson, L. and Thorslund, M. (1991). The national context of social innovation—Sweden. In: Kraan, R.J., Baldock, J., Davies, B., Evers, A., Johansson, L., Knapen, M., Thorslund, M. and Tunissen, C. (Eds), *Care for the Elderly: Significant Innovations in Three European Countries.* Westview Press, Colorado, pp. 28–44.

Kuypers, J.A. and Bengtson, V.L. (1973). Social breakdown and competence. A model of normal aging. *Hum. Develop.*, **16**, 181–201.

Levi-Montalcini, R. (1964). The nerve growth factor. *Ann. N.Y. Acad. Sci.*, **113**, 149–168.

Mullan, M., Crawford, F., Axelman, K., Houlden, H., Lilius, L., Winblad, B. and Lannfelt, L. (1992). A pathogenic mutation for probable Alzheimer's disease in the APP gene at N-terminus of ß-amyloid. *Nature Gene.*, **1**, 345–347.

Nordberg, A., Lilja, A., Lundqvist, H., Hartvig, P., Amberla, K., Viitanen, M., Warpman, U., Johansson, M., Hellström-Lindahl, E., Bjurling, P., Fasth, K.J., Långström, B. and Winblad, B. (1992). Tacrine restores cholinergic nicotinic receptors and glucose metabolism in Alzheimer's patients as visualized by positron emission tomography. *Neurobiol. Aging*, **6**, 747–758.

Olson, L., Nordberg, A., von Holst, H., Bäckman, L., Ebendal, T., Alafuzoff, I., Amberla, K., Hatrvig, P., Herlitz, A., Lilja, A., Lundqvist, H., Långström, B., Meyerson, B., Persson, A., Viitanen, M., Winblad, B. and Seiger, å. (1992). Nerve growth factor affects ^{11}C-nicotine binding, blood flow, EEG, and verbal episodic memory in an Alzheimer patient (Case report). *J. Neural Tramsm.*, **4**, 79–95.

Preston, G.A.N. (1986). Dementia in elderly adults: prevalence and institutionalization. *J. Gerontol.*, **41**, 261–267.

Sandman, P.O. (1990). Is good care the best treatment for the Alzheimer patient? *Acta Neurol. Scand.*, **129** (Suppl. 82), 37–39.

Stoller, E.P. and Pugliesi, K.L. (1988). Informal networks of community-based elderly. *Res. Aging*, **10**, 499–516.

IV

The Social Impact
of Alzheimer's Disease

The Management of Alzheimer's Disease
Edited by Gordon K. Wilcock
©1993 Wrightson Biomedical Publishing Ltd

11

Care for the Carers:
The Role of Respite Services

ENID LEVIN

Research Unit, National Institute for Social Work, London, UK

INTRODUCTION

The preceding chapters have provided a comprehensive account of advances in basic scientific research and clinical practice. By contrast, this chapter focuses on the experiences of thousands of ordinary people who cope daily with the consequences of Alzheimer's disease and on the care services potentially available to help them.

As earlier contributors of this book have stated, in almost every country family members, usually very close kin and usually women, play a major part in the care of people with dementia. Despite wide variations in the organization, level and mix of community and residential services, most governments pursue the policy of home-based care for very dependent people (Keen, 1992). As a result, in rhetoric if not in reality, they have begun to attach importance to providing services to the carers upon whom the success of community care largely depends. Thus in the United Kingdom developing respite services is one of the government's key objectives for service delivery at a time of major changes in the arrangements for community care and the financing of residential care (Secretaries of State, 1989; The NHS and Community Care Act 1990). In Australia, the National Action Plan for Dementia Care (Commonwealth Department of Health, 1992) recommends additional resources for respite care as part of the policy to encourage the development of such provision.

Some readers may attribute the increasing emphasis on home-based care and support for carers to the escalating costs of publicly funded residential care in the present economic climate and to the belief that community care is the cheaper option. Others may prefer to think that it is driven by notions

119

of social justice and by responsiveness to the pressure from Alzheimer's Disease Societies and the information provided by systematic research. Whatever the reasons for the policy, the development of services for carers— or as a minimum requirement, the preservation of existing levels of service— commands broad public support and is in keeping with the preferences of elderly people and many carers (Sinclair *et al.*, 1990).

However, there is rather less agreement about the aims of these services, the form that they should take and the criteria to be used in assessing their effectiveness. Some researchers (Brodaty and Gresham, 1992; Nolan and Grant, 1992) have pointed out that the emphasis on respite services rests on the implicit assumption that some time off will reduce the level of distress in a carer and that, in turn, this will delay the entry of the person with dementia into permanent care. Others (Levin *et al.*, 1989; Levin and Moriarty, 1990; O'Connor *et al.*, 1991; Wells *et al.*, 1990) have suggested that it is important to clarify whether the primary aim of respite services is to assist those who want to care for as long as they wish to do so or whether it is to ration, postpone or substitute for residential care, whatever the personal costs to the primary carers. These researchers have raised issues about the place of respite care in the wider spectrum of services, its effects on elderly people and their carers, its limits and the scope for expansion and improvements in existing services. They leave us in no doubt, however, about the key contribution of comprehensive services to the management of Alzheimer's disease at home. In this chapter, therefore, I will present some findings from recently completed research (Levin *et al.*, 1992) on packages of respite care, drawing out the implications for carers and elderly people with dementia on the one hand and for those who plan, purchase, provide and evaluate services on the other. Before introducing the study, I will set out some of the reasons for singling out the carers of dementia sufferers as a group whose needs for services require special attention and then identify the range of services encompassed by the word 'respite'.

THE CASE FOR SUPPORT TO CARERS

Reasons for treating the carers of people with Alzheimer's disease and related disorders as a priority group for services are described in the following sections.

Population changes and the age-related nature of dementia

As Copeland shows in Chapter 1, in Great Britain it is estimated that the number of people aged 85 years and over will continue to rise rapidly in the next decade. The prevalence rate of dementia doubles with each additional

5.1 years of age, reaching about 20% in the case of those aged 85–89. In consequence, it is expected that care will have to be provided for a growing number of very elderly people with moderate and severe dementia.

Use of services

It is important to remember that elderly people with dementia are far more likely than others to enter permanent residential care. In general, the proportion of all sufferers who live in residential care increases with the severity of the degree of dementia. Studies in Europe, North America and Australia estimate that about 50% of elderly people who live in residential care have dementing illnesses (Sinclair *et al.*, 1990; Gilleard, 1992; Brodaty and Gresham, 1992).

Recent research confirms also that elderly people with dementia make heavier use of a range of community services, those with moderate and severe dementia being particularly likely to use two or more community services (O'Connor *et al.*, 1989; Livingston *et al.*, 1990). Yet many of those using community services require additional support and many others do not receive relevant services at all (Levin *et al.*, 1989, 1992).

Strain on carers

Within the community, most people with moderate or severe dementia are cared for by a spouse or a child in the same household (Twigg, 1992). The problems and stresses experienced by these main carers are now so well documented that Zarit (1989) has argued that they do not require further study. Importantly, it has been shown that, in general, caring for someone with dementia is more stressful than caring for someone with a physical disability (Noelker and Poulshock, 1982; O'Connor *et al.*, 1990). For example, in their Cambridge community survey, O'Connor *et al.* (1990) found that the carers coping with dementia reported more problems, greater problem severity, and greater strain than other carers, and that problems and strain increased with the degree of dementia. As studies of carers known to services have shown, disturbed behaviours and relationships are poorly tolerated (Levin *et al.*, 1989). This led Briggs to suggest in Chapter 5 that greater professional effort should be devoted to helping carers to cope with these distressing problems.

Impact of services

While research has paid far more attention to the stresses on carers (Morris *et al.*, 1988) than to the interventions which might alleviate them, a small but growing number of studies are beginning to assess the effects of services.

Strikingly, six studies (Challis *et al.*, 1988; Gibbins, 1986; Gilleard, 1987; Levin *et al.*, 1989, 1992; Wells *et al.*, 1990) have shown that, when standard services only are provided, the mental health of those caring for very dependent people improves, on average, if their dependent enters residential care. By contrast, the mental health of those who continue to provide care shows, on average, no such sign of improvement. On this evidence, then, permanent residential care for people with dementia is one service which generally reduces the level of strain on carers. Therefore, a key question is whether community services can be as beneficial. On this matter, the conclusions from research are equivocal and many more studies evaluating the effects of various types, amounts and combinations of services on particular groups of carers and elderly people are required.

A useful start in this direction has been made by studies of new approaches to delivering services (Askham and Thompson, 1990; Donaldson *et al.*, 1988; Thornton, 1988) and new intervention programmes, such as education and training for carers (Ehrlich and White, 1991). Others have examined the effects of either one type of service, such as day care or relief admissions to homes or hospitals (Berry *et al.*, 1991; Brodaty and Gresham, 1992; Burdz *et al.*, 1988; Gilleard, 1987; Nolan and Grant, 1992; Wells *et al.*, 1990; Wimo *et al.*, 1992) or combinations of various services (Lawton *et al.*, 1989; Levin *et al.*, 1989, 1992; Montgomery and Borgatta, 1989). In an experimental study of over 500 carers, Montgomery and Borgatta found that a combination of respite and educational services was particularly effective in helping adult children to delay placement of a parent in residential care. Using a different type of comparative approach, the first National Institute for Social Work (NISW) study found that home help, community nursing and day care, especially in combination, had beneficial effects on some carers' mental health; however, relief care in homes and hospitals increased the likelihood of an elderly person's admission to permanent residential care (Levin *et al.*, 1989).

Findings from the recently completed NISW study, which focused upon respite services for carers living with a confused elderly person are reported in the rest of this chapter.

WHAT ARE RESPITE SERVICES?

The word 'respite' must be defined because it has come to have more than one meaning when used to describe services. For example, it sometimes refers only to short stays in residential care. Increasingly, it is used, as I am using it, to refer to any service which gives carers a temporary break from their care-giving responsibilities. Thus it covers services provided within the home—sitting, carers' support and in-home respite—and services outside the home—day care and relief care in residential homes, hospitals and family settings. An individual carer may use only one form of respite or their 'package' may be made up of a combination of services. Respite services in any one area may be provided by health, social services and the independent sector.

THE NISW STUDY

Funded by the Department of Health, our research was undertaken in collaboration with health, social services and voluntary organizations in three areas: a city in the north of England, a city in the south, and a rural area in the Midlands. As a first step, in each area the arrangers and providers of respite care across these agencies completed forms providing details on each confused person aged 65 or over and living with at least one other person who was using their service on a given date. A random sample of elderly people and their carers was drawn from the forms completed on 528 people. Two hundred and eighty-seven carers and the person whom they looked after were interviewed. About one year later, we established outcomes for the 287 elderly people in terms of whether they were at home, had died or entered residential care. Two hundred and forty three carers were reinterviewed.

The research provides detailed information on the users of different types and combinations of day, sitting and relief care services and on the carers' experiences and views of the services. It examines the effectiveness of differing mixes of respite services in terms of their acceptability to carers and their impact on the carer's mental health and on the elderly people themselves. In the conclusions to our research report (Levin *et al.*, 1992), we discuss the scope for developing and improving local respite services.

The elderly people

Given earlier work, we were not surprised that the 287 people in the study formed a very elderly, heavily dependent group. The mean age of people in the sample was 79.1 years and a quarter of them were aged 85–98. Women outnumbered men by a ratio of 3:2. Almost all the men, but less than half the women, were still married.

The Memory and Information Section of the Clifton Assessment Procedure for the Elderly (CAPE) (Pattie and Gilleard, 1979) was one of the measures used to assess each elderly person's mental state. At first interview, the scores on the CAPE suggested that three in five people were markedly or severely cognitively impaired and a further one in five was moderately impaired. Of course, many of these elderly people had more than one health problem which interfered in some instances with their everyday activities. Arthritis was the most frequently reported condition. An overall rating of degree of dependency was provided by the elderly people's scores on the Behaviour Rating Scale of the CAPE, which was completed by their carers; on this basis, almost three-quarters were classified as highly or maximally dependent. In the year between interviews, the abilities of most elderly people deteriorated and their carers faced increasing pressure. As can be seen, many elderly people in this group using respite services were as seriously incapacitated as those in residential care.

The carers

The study confirmed that in practice it is very close kin who are responsible for providing community care for people with moderate or severe dementia. The 287 carers were: wives (33%), husbands (24%), daughters (22%), sons (6%), daughters-in-law (6%), siblings (5%) and others (4%). The vast majority (85%) were spouses or children.

Overall, seven in 10 carers were women; however, among the important sub-group formed by elderly carers, men, nearly all husbands, did not outnumber women greatly. The mean age of the carers was 66 years and over 40% reported having a longstanding illness or disability. The amount of help given to the elderly person by their carer usually outstripped that given by other people.

Two in three carers and elderly people had lived together for more than 25 years and, although they had a heavy workload and many other difficulties, most carers wanted this arrangement to continue. At first interview and consistent with other studies (Sinclair et al., 1990), only 11% of the carers said they would definitely accept residential care; by contrast, 61% of the carers said they would definitely refuse it.

Despite their willingness to care, there was evidence that the strain on some carers was great. The carers completed the 28-point General Health Questionnaire (GHQ) (Goldberg and Williams, 1988) and the Selfcare (D) (Bird et al., 1987) at both interviews so that we had a means of assessing their mental health and the impact of caring upon it. As indicated by the initial Selfcare (D) scores, 27% of carers were likely to have a depressive illness. In the case of the GHQ, which is a widely used screening test for identifying non-psychotic psychiatric illness, scores of six or over were recorded for two in five carers, suggesting a high level of psychological strain.

Female carers had higher GHQ scores, on average, than male carers and female and male carers with physical disabilities and longstanding illnesses had higher GHQ scores, on average, than others. The combination of factors associated with GHQ scores included gender of the carer, their physical health, and the number and nature of the precise problems faced in caregiving. Thus the higher the level of dependency and the greater the behavioural disturbance in the elderly people, the higher the carers' GHQ scores.

The sources and nature of stresses on the carers were: *practical*—giving the elderly people regular help with many aspects of their personal care; *behavioural*—for example incontinence, unsafe acts and night disturbance; *interpersonal*—for example, sadness at the change in their relatives and losing their tempers with them; and *social*—restrictions on getting out, leisure time and visiting family and friends.

Once these problems have been identified by thorough assessment, many can be alleviated, if not eliminated, by practical, professional and other forms of help. Clearly, respite services are relevant to the restrictions on social life which arise from caring and to the carers' needs to take a break. The carers and elderly people in our sample spent, on average, 16 hours apart in a typical week. Half the carers never left their relatives alone in the house and one-third thought that they spent too much time together. Ninety per cent of the carers considered that they were restricted to some extent by caring, nearly half of them very much so. Their reactions to this difficulty varied, but those who did not find it bothersome were a minority group. Against this background, the strengths, limitations and potential current respite services can be assessed.

The services

In each of three study areas a wide range of agencies and professions contributed to the organization, funding and delivery of respite services. Some of their contributions were unique, some were complementary and others overlapped or substituted for each other. For example, day care was obtained through the National Health Service, social services, voluntary organizations and, albeit rarely, the private sector. An individual carer's respite service might be made up of a sitter visiting from a voluntary organization, day care for the elderly person in a social services centre and residential relief care in a hospital. This pattern has resulted in part from the gradual evolution of services over the years with one agency attempting, for example, to meet a gap or shortfall in the provision of others or obtaining funding for a new initiative. Now health and social services are required to act jointly in collaboration with the voluntary and private sectors to develop locality services and programmes of care for individuals. Our study identified a range of issues which merit the attention of health and social care planners, purchasers and providers and provided information relevant to their task.

Variation

The capacity of services to assist carers is limited by the level and type of local provision. There were major variations between the three areas in the overall resources allocated to respite, in the balance of the contributions from the various sectors and in the availability of new kinds of services. In consequence, the package of respite which can be arranged for carers in one locality cannot necessarily be arranged for those with similar problems in others. For example, while day care and residential relief care are available from some source in most areas, sitting and family-based relief care schemes are patchily available within areas and across the country. Sitting services were more extensive in one study area than those in the other two. Thus the package of respite and its sources depended partly upon where the carer lived.

Packages of respite

Most carers used a combination of two or three types of respite service. Of those with respite in our sample, 34% used either day care or sitting or relief care, 50% used two of these services and 16% used all three of them. Day care was the main source of a break during the week; relief care in a home or a hospital was used very infrequently on its own. The commonest package was made up of day care combined with relief care. The package of respite which included residential relief care was targeted at the carers who showed signs of psychological strain, and at those whose elderly relatives were severely dependent and who manifested the highest number of major behavioural and interpersonal problems. Moreover, once the carers had accepted respite services, most continued to use them for as long as those they cared for remained at home: the main reasons for ceasing to use the services between first and second interviews were that an elderly person had died or entered permanent residential care.

Whilst giving the more intensive packages of respite to the most severely dependent and behaviourally disturbed people is in accordance with the official policy of targeting services at 'those in greatest need' (Secretaries of State, 1989), it limits the scope for using services with the intention of preventing strain in carers and for giving the carers the opportunity to choose which respite services they would like.

Amount and timing of services

A key task for care managers is to construct service packages which are responsive to the individual, differing and changing needs of carers and their dependants. On our evidence, expansion and changes in the services will be necessary if this objective is to be achieved.

Usually, respite services had been allocated to the carers in standard amounts and at standard intervals. Thus the elderly people with day care attended once a week, on average, in one area and twice a week in the other two areas. Overall, carers with sitters were visited once or twice a week, and the sitter spent about three and a half hours per week, on average, with the elderly people; in one area, however, the majority of those with sitters had a weekly service of over five hours. In each area, regular residential respite was offered to most carers in inflexible blocks of two weeks, with intervals of six, eight or 12 weeks between breaks. The times of the day and days of the week that services were available were somewhat standard: day care on weekdays between the hours of 10 a.m. and 3.30 p.m. and rarely at weekends; sitting in the mornings or afternoons, infrequently in the evenings and again, rarely at weekends; relief care for a fortnight or a week with the stay beginning and ending on a Saturday. The carers fitted in with the service. For example, they appreciated that day care could not be offered in a particular unit on a Wednesday if the unit only catered for people with dementia on a Tuesday. However, it was not surprising that some carers would have liked the service at different times of the day or the week and some would have liked a more frequent service. Therefore we would suggest that priority should be accorded to expanding and extending these services so that they may address the carer's requirements more efficiently.

Carers' views

The carers' task was unremitting in that people with dementia may be very difficult to live with and very difficult to leave on their own. The carers' opinions on the role of services in their lives should be assessed in the context of the limited support available from other sources. Consistent with the findings of many other studies (Sinclair *et al.*, 1990; Twigg, 1992), we found the most carers in our sample had relatives and friends who visited, telphoned and, at times, gave some practical help; but many did not have family and friends who were able and willing to attend to the elderly person: less than half the carers said that a relative or friend had looked after the elderly person for a few hours during the day, and only 11% said that someone had taken over from them for at least 24 hours in the previous year. Thus, many carers in this study had to rely heavily on services for a break. The strong link between the hours the elderly people went to day care and the total number of hours that they were apart from their carers each week highlights this reliance.

Therefore, it was not surprising that the *carers with respite services valued them highly* and could identify improvements in their own life on acceptance of respite. Indeed, half of those with the regular break afforded by day care or sitting thought that these services improved their lives greatly. For example, assessing the advantages of day care, one carer said, 'I'd go mad if I didn't have a day to myself'; assessing the impact of a sitting service once a week, another said, 'It's made a world of difference. It gives me something to look forward to each week'; and talking about residential respite, a husband said, 'It's taken a lot of worry off my mind now she goes every six weeks'.

The carers could be very specific about the kinds of things which respite services enabled them to do. Most mentioned a range of benefits accruing from the service, such as having some time to themselves, being able to visit friends and get on with the chores. However, it was striking that the activities mentioned most frequently were essential, everyday tasks such as shopping, paying the bills and going to the hairdressers. For example, two-thirds of those with day care and half of those with sitting said that the services enabled them to do the shopping, whilst the proportion mentioning that it enabled them to pursue their leisure activities fell in both cases to about one-third.

Most carers using sitting or day care thought that their elderly relative derived some direct benefit from the service also. One daughter's opinion of the benefit of day care to her mother was, 'She seems a little more alert the next day. She talks a lot more'. A husband said of the sitter's visit, 'It's someone different who will talk to her and listen'. The carer's opinions about the effects of residential respite on the elderly people were more divided. When compared with their views about the other two respite services, the carers were much more likely to say that their relatives did not benefit from residential relief care. Overall, about two in five carers felt that relief care breaks had no effect, either beneficial or detrimental, upon the elderly person. As one carer put it, 'Nothing changed at all, it was as though he hadn't been away'. However, it was noteworthy that almost one-third of carers saw an improvement in their relative after relief care and that only 11% reported a deterioration in their relative; the remaining minority thought that the overall effect of relief care was mixed.

Researchers and others who evaluate and monitor services generally take account of the carers' and users' views but do not regard them as sufficient in themselves to make the case for providing services. Typically, the carers in our sample were very positive about the services. They were looking after elderly people who could not manage without their help and I would suggest that their views on the benefits of the services should be listened to carefully and taken very seriously. So too, should their views on the changes that they would like to see in the services, for the carers were very realistic also about the limitations of services and identified between them many areas for improvement in practice. Respite services given in standard amounts and at standard times did not necessarily remove the restrictions of caring. A key question is whether this problem might be alleviated by tackling the restrictions most keenly felt: after all, a sitting service for two hours on a Tuesday may be useful in itself but will not enable a carer to continue to play golf with friends on Wednesday or attend a funeral at short notice on Friday.

Effects of services

On follow-up of the 287 elderly people about one year later, 46% were living at home, 19% were in residential care and 35% had died. It was striking that of the survivors, 72% were still at home.

Our findings confirmed the essential contribution of resident carers to community care. First, of the carers, 7% were known to have died or to have entered residential care; only one of the elderly dependents of this group remained at home which suggested that the carers were almost always irreplaceable. Secondly, of the elderly people who were no longer at home, six in 10 had died; thus the carers had looked after most of this group until the last few weeks or months of their lives. Thirdly, attributes of the carers at first interview influenced whether the elderly people were at home or in residential care on follow-up. The likelihood of entry into residential care was affected by a combination of factors. These included the carers' attitudes to continuing to care and their mental health at first interview, the severity of cognitive impairment in the elderly people and the degree to which their dependency increased between first interview and last month at home, and the use of residential relief care. However, our analysis has shown that of the factors predicting admission, the carer's wish for permanent residential care for an elderly person at first interview was by far the most important.

Overall, elderly people who had residential relief care were more likely to enter permanent residential care than others. However, it was striking that two-thirds of the survivors who used residential relief care at first interview were at home on follow-up. Moreover, the greater the number of months since a carer had first used residential relief care, the greater the likelihood that an elderly person was at home.

As Brodaty and Gresham (1992) have shown, the balance of evidence from research refutes the suggestion that people going into residential respite die earlier. Our study provides additional evidence which supports this statement: as found in the first NISW study (Levin *et al.*, 1989), elderly people who entered residential respite were no more likely than others to have died.

Finally, we turn to the question of whether respite services had a detectable impact on the carers' mental health. As stated earlier in this chapter, our study added to the small but increasing number of studies which have shown that the mental health of the carers improves, on average, if their dependant enters permanent residential care; by contrast, the mental health of those who continue to provide care shows no such signs of improvement. We find it unsurprising that we were unable to detect beneficial effects of respite services on the carers' mental health: in our view, this result should be interpreted in the context of the heavy dependency of many elderly people, the deterioration in their abilities after first interview, the complex factors which contribute to the level of strain in the carers and the limited amount of respite provided by the standard community services.

CONCLUSIONS

Our study confirmed that the carers who used respite services were looking after a group of very dependent elderly people, many of whom were as seriously incapacitated as those in residential care. The carers were very close kin, often elderly themselves and most wanted to continue to provide care as long as they were able. On our evidence, their contribution to the care of their elderly relatives was essential and almost always irreplaceable. The carers' task was unremitting and could be very stressful and, as their relatives deteriorated, they faced increasing pressure. Each carer was unique and their needs to take a break changed over time; therefore, there was no single type and level of respite which would have suited all of them. It is against this background that the role of respite services should be assessed.

As shown, the carers' comments left us in no doubt about the positive contribution which respite services made to their lives. They valued these services highly and found them relevant to many, if not all, the problems they faced. However, respite services at their current levels could not remove entirely the restrictions imposed by caring. For the carers in this sample, a package of respite made up of day care twice a day, sitting services once a week and relief care for a fortnight in every eight weeks was intensive; it was targeted at carers who showed signs of great strain and who were looking after the most heavily dependent people. If we see services as forming a continuum from permanent residential care at one end to no breaks for the carers at the other, then even the relatively intensive packages of respite given to the carers fall far short of the 'permanent care' end of the continuum in terms of relief afforded to the carers.

My colleagues and I would suggest, therefore, that current levels of provision put limits on the contribution of respite services to community care. The aims of these services have been widely debated. On our evidence, respite services continue to be used to serve three purposes: first, they are used to ration and postpone the use of permanent care which some carers, albeit a minority, would have preferred; secondly, they are used to prepare both the carer and the elderly person gradually for permanent care; and thirdly, they are used to support carers who want to continue to provide care. These services cannot substitute currently for permanent care; moreover, it would seem unreasonable to expect them to have a detectable impact on the carers' mental health. It may be realistic, therefore, to measure the usefulness of respite by assessing the extent to which it alleviates the precise problems the carers face. Now the challenge lies in ensuring that respite services have the resources and standards of practice to respond flexibly to the carers' varying and changing requirements.

REFERENCES

Askham, J. and Thompson, C. (1990). *Dementia and Home Care: A Research Report on a Home Support Scheme for Dementia Sufferers.* Age Concern, Mitcham.

Berry, G.L., Zarit, S.H. and Rabatin, V.X. (1991). Caregiver activity on respite and non respite days: a comparison of two service approaches. *Gerontologist*, **31**, 830–835.

Bird, A.S., Macdonald, A.J.D., Mann, A.H. and Philpott, M.P. (1987). Preliminary experience with the Selfcare (D): a self-rating depression questionnaire for use in elderly, non-institutionalised subjects. *Int. J. Geriatr. Psychiatry*, **2**, 31–38.

Brodaty, H. and Gresham, M. (1992). Prescribing residential respite care for dementia-effects, side-effects, indications and dosage. *Int. J. Geriatr. Psychiatry*, **7**, 357–362.

Burdz, M.P., Eaton, W.O. and Bond, J.B. (1988). Effects of respite care on dementia and non dementia patients and their caregivers. *Psychol. Aging*, **3**, 38–42.

Challis, D., Chessum, R., Chesterman, J., Luckett, R. and Woods, B. (1988). Community care for the frail elderly: an urban experiment. *Br. J. Soc. Work*, **18** (Suppl.) 13–41

Commonwealth Department of Health, Housing and Community Services (1992). *National Action Plan for Dementia Care.* Australian Government Publishing Service, Canberra.

Donaldson, C., Clark, K., Gregson, B., Backhouse, M. and Pragnall, C. (1988). *Evaluation of a Family Support Unit for Elderly Mentally Infirm People and their Carers.* Health Care Research Unit Report 34, University of Newcastle upon Tyne.

Ehrlich, P. and White, J. (1991). TOPS: a consumer approach to Alzheimer's respite programs. *Gerontologist*, **31**, 686–691.

Gibbins, R. (1986). *Oundle Community Care Unit: An Evaluation of an Initiative in the Care of the Elderly Mentally Infirm.* Northamptonshire County Council, Northampton.

Gilleard, C.J. (1987). Influence of emotional distress among supporters on the outcome of psychogeriatric day care. *Br. J. Psychiatry*, **150**, 219–223.

Gilleard, C. (1992). Community care services for the elderly mentally infirm. In: Jones, G.M.M. and Miesen, B.M.L. (Eds), *Care-giving in Dementia: Research and Applications.* Tavistock/Routledge, London, pp. 293–313.

Goldberg, D. and Williams, P. (1988). *A User's Guide to the General Health Questionnaire.* NFER–Nelson Publishing Company, Windsor.

Keen, J. (1992). *Dementia.* Office of Health Economics, London.

Lawton, M.P., Brody, E.M. and Saperstein, A.R. (1989). A controlled study of respite service for caregivers of Alzheimer's patients. *Gerontologist*, **29**, 8–16.

Levin, E. and Moriarty, J. (1990). *'Ready to Cope Again': Sitting, Day and Relief Care for Carers of Confused Elderly People.* National Institute for Social Work, London.

Levin, E., Sinclair, I. and Gorbach, P. (1989). *Families, Services and Confusion in Old Age.* Avebury, Aldershot.

Levin, E., Moriarty, J. and Gorbach, P. (1992). *'I couldn't manage without the breaks': Respite Services for the Carers of Confused Elderly People.* Report to the Department of Health, National Institute for Social Work, London.

Livingston, G., Thomas, A., Graham, N., Blizard, B. and Mann, A. (1990). The Gospel Oak Project: the use of health and social services by dependent elderly people in the community. *Health Trends*, **22**, 70–73.

Montgomery, R.J.V. and Borgatta, E.F. (1989). The effects of alternative support strategies on family caregiving. *Gerontologist*, **29**, 457–464.

Morris, R.G., Morris, L.W. and Britton, P.G. (1988). Factors affecting the emotional wellbeing of the caregivers of dementia sufferers. *Br. J. Psychiatry*, **153**, 147–156.

Noelker, L.S. and Poulshock, S.W. (1982). *The Effects on Families of Caring for Impaired Elderly in Residence*. Benjamin Rose Institute, Cleveland.

Nolan, M. and Grant, G. (1992). *Regular Respite: An Evaluation of a Hospital Rota Bed Scheme for Elderly People*. ACE Books, Age Concern, London.

O'Connor, D.W., Pollitt, P.A., Brook, C.P.B. and Reiss, B.B. (1989). The distribution of services to demented elderly people living in the community. *Int. J. Geriatr. Psychiatry*, **4**, 339–344.

O'Connor, D.W., Pollitt, P.A., Roth, M., Brook, C.P.B. and Reiss, B.B. (1990). Problems reported by relatives in a community study of dementia. *Br. J. Psychiatry*, **156**, 835–841.

O'Connor, D.W., Pollitt, P.A., Brook, C.P.B., Reiss, B.B. and Roth, M. (1991). Does early intervention reduce the number of elderly people with dementia admitted to institutions for long-term care? *Br. Med. J.*, **302**, 871–875.

Pattie, A.H. and Gilleard, C.J. (1979). *Manual of the Clifton Assessment Procedure for the Elderly*. Hodder and Stoughton, Kent.

Secretaries of State for Health, Social Security, Scotland and Wales. (1989). *Caring for People: Community Care in the Next Decade and Beyond*. CM 849, HMSO, London.

Sinclair, L., Parker, R., Leat, D. and Williams, J. (1990). *The Kaleidoscope of Care: a Review of Research on Welfare Provision for Elderly People*. HMSO, London.

The National Health Service and Community Care Act (1990). HMSO, London.

Thornton, P. (1988). *Creating a Break: a Home Care Relief Scheme for Elderly People and their Supporters*. Age Concern, Mitcham.

Twigg, J. (Ed.) (1992). *Carers: Research and Practice*. HMSO, London.

Wells, Y.D., Jorm, A.F., Jordan, F. and Lefroy, D. (1990). Effects on care-givers of special day care programmes for dementia sufferers. *Aust. N.Z. J. Psychiatry*, **24**, 1–9.

Wimo, A., Wallin, J., Lungren, K., Rönnback, E., Asplund, K., Mattson, B. and Krakau, I. (1990). Impact of day care on dementia patients—costs, wellbeing and relatives' views. *Family Practice*, **7**, 279–286.

Zarit, S. (1989). Do we need another stress and caregiving study? *Gerontologist*, **29**, 147.

The Management of Alzheimer's Disease
Edited by Gordon K. Wilcock
©1993 Wrightson Biomedical Publishing Ltd

12

Home from Home:
Practical Aspects of Caring for the
Elderly Confused in a Nursing Home

CAROLINE REEVES

Manager, St George's Nursing Home, Cobham, UK

CREATING THE RIGHT ENVIRONMENT

The obvious first point to make is that every nursing home is different. Each has its own layout and facilities, its own philosophies and its own style of management. Most importantly, each home has a unique blend of personalities and skills amongst its staff. To date there has been little research on the relationship between the confused and their environments, but it is recognized that a welcoming, familiar environment has good results, particularly where residents have choice, freedom and activity.

There has been much debate about the subject of segregation. Whilst some feel that integration is the best policy for reasons of normalization, it should be remembered that this is difficult for residents who are not confused; these residents may feel distressed at listening to repetitive and senseless talk, seeing their possessions disappear and watching restlessness, agitation and socially unacceptable behaviour. Thus segregation can be hugely advantageous if the environment and facilities of the home can be designed to suit the cognitive limitations of the confused. However, it is well recognized that the number of people suffering from Alzheimer's disease and other dementias has increased dramatically and will continue to do so. Over the next few years, there may be rapid growth in the number of homes caring for the confused, and the debate about segregation may be less relevant.

DESIGN FEATURES

Henderson (1980) suggested some useful design features which might be incorporated into a home for the confused.

- The accommodation should create a homely welcoming atmosphere, and provide a safe and secure place for the resident to live. Single-storey buildings are ideal, because the likelihood of falls is considerably decreased. This layout also enables much better supervision. A proven effective design is the cross-shaped building used by several modern homes. There are few hidden corners, and it is very difficult for a resident to wander out of sight of staff.
- On the other hand, the desire to wander must be catered for. Open spaces which are easily accessible from bedrooms and lounges give a sense of freedom. Circular return routes rather than corridors which lead to dead ends reduce frustration and aggression.
- The gardens too should have circular paths which are flat but interesting: statuary, seats and bird tables all add to the environment. The use of long-established flowers such as roses can be very helpful: many elderly people will remember a rose bush which has been a part of their environment for many years. The sound of running water is therapeutic, and safely enclosed fountains and ponds are often appreciated. Well planned gardens can help to overcome the institutional nature of the home; the use of a densely grown rhododendron looks far less institutional than security fencing whilst still containing the ardent wanderer.
- Residents like to have familiar personal items around them, such as pictures, a particular chair or a table. These provide feelings of security. The arrangement of free-standing furniture to the resident's own tastes can aid the settling-in process.
- Bedroom doors and toilets should be clearly signposted, graphically where possible. Good lighting is essential as illusions can result from dimly lit corridors and bedrooms: for example, whilst dressing one morning with only the bedside light on, one of my residents thought that a stocking on the floor was a snake. She left the room shrieking, and it took some time to pacify her.

In addition, the following points are important.

- It is essential that we provide a safe environment, so that residents are unable to leave the home without supervision. If exits are not too highly visible, the desire to leave will not be stimulated. Whilst 'Exit' fire signs are a legal requirement, 'Way Out' signs can create feelings of entrapment. Similarly, the ostentatious use of keys or the use of only one exit door can create the desire to leave. There is much debate as to the best way of managing this desire whilst trying to maintain the resident's dignity. Some psychiatric units use two-handled baffle locks and electronic tagging; these are hardly dignified, and given the right environment and management should not be necessary. I have personally found digital locks with a short code preferable as they are quick for staff to use and you do not find people pulling at door handles struggling to get out.

- If space is available, hairdressing should be undertaken in a properly set up salon; similar principles apply to facilities for medical consultations and chiropody. The proper use of rooms will not contribute to the confusion: on the contrary, residents will feel that they are 'going out' to these places, and may be reminded of earlier experiences. Moreover, residents will be encouraged to use the services available to them.
- Many people suffering from confusion will be unable to communicate directly that the environment is uncomfortable to them; their discomfort may be shown in other ways, such as restlessness, irritability and aggression. Heating should be variable so that rooms can be heated to the different levels required by residents. Good ventilation and the use of dimmer switches can help to make an environment more comfortable.
- Seating in shared areas should not be arranged in institutional straight lines around the room, but in small circular groups to encourage conversation.
- Caring for the confused is a stressful job, and staff must be properly looked after. There must be a comfortable staff room away from residents' living areas so that they can unwind. If managers cannot look after their staff, they are unlikely to be sensitive to the needs of the more vulnerable people in their care.

NURSING CARE

Primary nursing

Under the primary nursing system, nurses work in teams and are assigned to particular residents. For example, in my home three teams of 12 covering a 24 hour period are assigned to 40 residents. It is my experience that the confused respond extremely well to familiar faces and are able to recognize and build relationships with staff who care for them daily on an ongoing basis. Very often even the most confused residents will respond to 'their' nurses, but not to a nurse they do not know well.

A qualified nurse leads each team, prescribing the care for the assigned residents in consultation with all the team members. I have also included the domestic team as they have direct daily contact with residents when cleaning their rooms and doing the laundry. It gives them the feeling that they are part of the team providing care, rather than working in isolation. Primary nursing is also more efficient, because the team knows the individual needs of each resident. For example in my home Mrs P. will not have a bath at all, but will have a good strip wash in the morning and before going to bed. Knowing this, the staff will avoid causing distress by forcing her to bath against her will.

Individual care plans

These are a vital component of primary care. Because every resident is unique and has different needs, all residents should have an individual and practical care plan for the nursing team to follow. This must include:

- a baseline assessment on admission,
- a detailed but simple plan of action in relation to needs and problems,
- a review section,
- day to day notes.

The baseline assessment considers the apparent physical, mental and social needs, strengths, weaknesses and preferences of the resident. This should always be done with the assistance of the relatives, close friends, specialists and of course the person who is receiving the care whenever possible, over a period of a week or two. The observations of nursing staff should also be included. Then the plan of action tailored to each person's need can be drawn up. For example, Mr W. wanders incessantly in the evenings. If he is taken out for a short walk at about 3 p.m. this is generally curtailed. If it is not, he is taken out for another walk at 6 p.m. The plan of action must be described in easy to follow instructions, and should contain a range of options. The condition of residents will change over time; regular review is therefore an essential part of the care plan. Day to day notes are taken in order to monitor residents' well-being, and to provide a means of communication for other members of staff.

One may argue that as Alzheimer's disease is an on-going progressive condition with no imminent hope of a cure, then is it necessary to spend precious time on paperwork and is it not quicker to organize care on a task orientated basis and plan all activities in groups? It probably would be, but we would be operating a system of care which does not view people as individuals with unique needs and benefitting from a tailor-made plan of care. Also staff will have a greater degree of satisfaction and a more positive approach to the needs of residents if they feel they are giving personalized attention and relate to residents as a person.

Care should be flexible, partly to recognize residents' individuality and party because of the hourly or daily changes in mood which are created by the progressive dementias. The provision of choice of dress, bed times, visiting times and activities are instrumental in preventing passivity, withdrawal and apathy. To give residents a degree of choice is to make us responsive to their needs, rather than to mould their routines to an institutional format. This also frees staff rom the institutional routine; nurses feel that they are providing real care, and morale is improved accordingly.

DAY TO DAY CARE

To put into practice these principles regarding individuality, a display book can be created for each resident. I use the title 'This is Your Life'; the display book is completed with the help of residents and their relatives, and consists of information on background, family, likes and dislikes, hobbies and significant people in the resident's life—both past and present. It is important that we get the facts right so as not to add to the confusion. Old photographs, displayed in chronological order, together with photographs taken in the home, are used for the following reasons:

- they provide a spur to memory and reminiscence;
- relatives are assured that activities are taking place and that the resident is not merely sitting around all day;
- it is important that staff are persuaded to see residents as individuals with life stories, interests and aptitudes;
- photographs are a good aid to conversation between staff, relatives and residents;
- the display book is returned to the family after death as a memoir, so that the time spent in the nursing home can be seen as an active part of the life rather than a prelude to death.

One interesting example is that of Mrs P. We could not understand why this resident insisted on collecting the cups after tea every day; when we questioned relatives we found that Mrs P. had been a pub landlady for much of her life, and was in effect acting out her past. We saw the benefits of this behaviour and allowed it to continue.

We also encourage residents and their families to keep diaries. The small pocket diary which we give to the residents can be used to record visits, general family news and future events. This would normally be kept up-to-date by a relative. The relative's diary can serve a similar purpose to the display book; it serves as a reminder, when it is needed, that not all times have been bad, and that there have been times when the resident has been active, lucid, happy and sociable.

Bathing and personal hygiene

For some residents, the occasional reminder about bathing and washing, together with minimal supervision and help, is sufficient. However, others require total help. Using the baseline assessment, staff can establish a routine shortly after the resident moves into the home. This should be a routine which they can regard as their own; it should be based on their habits and wishes, rather than upon institutional practices. For example, if the resident is incontinent and usually baths once a week and washes regularly, this should be accepted.

If the resident's personal hygiene requires intervention, then confrontation should be avoided at all costs. Offering a limited degree of choice can be persuasive; for example asking the question 'When would you like to have a bath—this morning or this afternoon?' is preferable to the statement 'You could do with a bath' or 'I've run a bath for you'. Some confused people are terrified of a full bath of water, so that a good strip wash or a bath only half filled is sufficient. Bathrooms should be homely and warm and use pleasant smelling toiletries to make them more enticing. Some residents like to have a bath with minimal fuss so staff need to be efficient and have everything ready before starting. In such cases, pampering should be avoided. Bath aids such as hand rails and non-slip mats make bathing easier and safer for the resident, and can provide a greater degree of independence.

The care of hair, nails, and make-up should be done according to the resident's wishes; these are particularly personal aspects of care, and areas over which the resident will wish to retain control for as long as possible. I have seen nurses on psychogeriatric wards put ribbons in ladies' hair because they think they look appealing, even when this is clearly not what the resident would wish if they were able to express a choice. Staff should use positive praise wherever possible by telling residents how nice they look.

Dressing

Dressing is often seen as an invasion of privacy by the confused and can be a source of aggression. A few basic guidelines will minimise frustration:

- Staff need to feel that they have the time to do things so that they do not feel flustered. The clothes in the wardrobe should be limited so that layers and layers of clothes cannot be put on. Residents in my care have often put on their whole wardrobes in layers. It is a good idea to store sets of clothes separately. Clothes can be left out in the correct sequence to avoid a muddle.
- Night clothes can be put away before day clothes are made available.
- Clothes must be big enough, as frustration mounts when arms won't go through sleeves easily. Smooth running zips, velcro fastenings, tights instead of stockings and zip flies can all make life easier. Although slip-on shoes are easier to put on, lace-ups will stay on for much longer.
- When attempting to undress a resident in the evening, conflict can often be avoided by allowing the resident to sleep in their day clothes after attempts at persuasion have failed. They have usually forgotten the problem by the morning. The confused are at their most tired in the evenings and conflict may be the last straw.

Meals

The ability to manage food is usually one of the last skills lost. As the disease progresses however, meal times become more of a trial. Patients lose their manual dexterity, fiddle with food, put knives into their mouths, spill drinks and eventually stop using cutlery altogether and need help with drinking. This sense of meal times as a trial needs to be addressed. Creating a relaxed and sociable atmosphere tends to reduce stress levels for staff and patient, so that neither comes to regard meals as battles to be won. The following methods can contribute to this atmosphere.

- There should not be too many people in the same dining room or around the same table, so that noise can be reduced and conflicting demands on staff avoided.
- Those who need considerable help with feeding should be fed in the privacy of their own rooms in order to retain their dignity. In periods of lucidity, other residents may dwell on their own fate if they see other more confused residents being fed.
- Appropriate seating is vitally important; physical discomfort is not conducive to eating well.

Individual residents can be assisted as follows.

- A sense of order can be created by putting one course on the table at a time, using essential cutlery only. Cups and mugs should have sturdy large handles, and be only half-filled.
- Meat should be tender and bite sized. If food needs to be liquidized then each food should be done separately so that it looks appetizing.
- Some residents prefer to use their fingers rather than cutlery. Manageable finger foods such as potato parcels make things much easier and encourage independence.
- Many residents seem to develop a sweet tooth—this can be used as an incentive to eat a main course.
- The restless and incessant walker will need a high calorie intake; some need up to 5000 calories a day to maintain their present weight. *Ensure Plus*, a high-calorie supplement which can be obtained on prescription, is packaged in small cartons which can be drunk 'on the move'.

Toileting

A well-designed home will have clearly identified toilets which are close to hand, easily accessible and well lit, thus helping to keep incontinence under control. Obviously toilets must be clean and have hand rails and raised toilet seats for those that need them. Apart from the obvious need for sanitary conditions, this will also have the effect of encouraging the confused resident to visit the toilet as often as needed. Each resident should have an assessment on admission in order to assess their toileting needs.

COPING WITH DIFFICULT PROBLEMS

The behavioural approach

Although a behavioural method of care does not claim to eliminate a particular problem entirely, this approach may highlight a cause of the behaviour which can be addressed. A number of techniques can be used, often avoiding the use of medication. The behavioural approach is essentially descriptive and is based upon observation. It avoids judgements, connotation and the use of pejorative language. Table 1 gives some examples. Once the behaviour has been observed and recorded, attempts can be made to interpret it and understand its possible causes.

Table 1. The behavioural approach.

Instead of	Use
Mr T. is aggressive	Mr T. hits out with his hands when approached by male staff
Mrs C. is withdrawn	Mrs C. avoids eye contact when spoken to

Case study

Observed behaviour:
Mrs S. puts on layer upon layer of clothes every afternoon around tea-time. She refuses to take them off when asked to by staff, and becomes tearful.

Analysis and possible causes:
Mrs S. feels cold in the late afternoon.
She is bored.
She feels insecure.
She gets her clothes muddled in her room.
She is depressed.

Possible solutions:
Ensure that the heating is satisfactory.
Offer an activity.
Demonstrate reassurance: she is wanted and safe.

Reduce the clothing in the wardrobe.
Seek psychiatric help.

The next step is to formulate a detailed but simple plan to test out the range of hypotheses. We did this in the case of Mrs S., but none of the hypotheses proved to be correct. We spoke about the behaviour with Mrs S.'s daughter, who informed us that she had always visited her mother at the same time every afternoon before Mrs S. had been moved into the home. It became clear that Mrs S. was going through the process of preparing for the visit, and became distressed when the daughter did not arrive. The staff approach effectively dashed her hopes. Mrs S. could not communicate this verbally. We could now assure her that her daughter would visit whenever possible and provide an activity at the appropriate time. The aggression and distress in this case were eliminated without medication. This demonstrates the need for an open mind, since hypotheses will frequently be proved incorrect.

Birchmore and Clague (1983) reported that a very confused lady who frequently shouted out when nurses were busy responded to being allocated periods of one-to-one care throughout the day. This did not eliminate the problem entirely, but reduced the shouting considerably. The quality of her life had improved, if only by a small degree.

On-going review of the behaviour and any improvement or deterioration will help staff to address the problem in the long term, rather than assuming that a period of remission is the end of the matter.

The behavioural approach places great demands on the care-givers in terms of time and commitment, but does focus on the individual by trying to understand the resident in relation to his environment; behaviours can be related to people, objects and specific situations. This approach can be used successfully in addressing such behaviours as incontinence, inappropriate sexual behaviour, wandering and aggression.

Incontinence

This can be the most distressing part of caring for the confused and is often the deciding factor in bringing a relative into a nursing home (Argyll et al., 1985). Incontinence can be equally distressing for sufferer and carer, and can be especially difficult to cope with when the sufferer denies all knowledge of it and blames somebody else. Incontinence is often one aspect of the natural progression of Alzheimer's disease, but it is unwise to assume that this is always the case. On admission, it is important that all physical conditions are eliminated before attributing the incontinence to the confusion. Cystitis, urinary tract infections, constipation, uncontrolled diabetes, an enlarged prostate, vaginitis and certain medications are all possible causes.

Other factors should also be taken into account. Is the resident depressed? Does he appear to have lost his hope and self respect? Has there been a bereavement or change in family circumstances, such as a son or daughter moving away? Has the environment changed in any way—has a toilet been repainted in a different colour, making it unfamiliar?

Close but relaxed supervision is the most effective method of dealing with incontinence. Nurses should look for warning signs, such as:

- restlessness particularly after drinks and meals,
- fidgeting with clothes,
- a woman squatting down, lifting her skirt or sitting down on a waste paper bin.

Prevention is better than cure, and regular care according to the needs of the individual is better than haphazard emergency intervention. Two- to three-hourly toileting after meals and before bedtime is enough for most. It is very unfair to toilet people throughout the night, and the benefits of frequent waking to keep a resident dry for an extra couple of hours should be weighed against the benefits of a good night's sleep, particularly where night sedation is prescribed. There are environmental implications in our approach to incontinence:

- the use of round waste paper baskets without lids, round rugs, and buckets should be avoided, as they are often mistaken for toilets;
- whilst not reducing overall fluid intake during the day, the bulk of fluid might be given before 4 p.m. to reduce nocturnal incontinence;
- faecal smearing often results from the resident feeling blocked and removing manually—it may be that the resident needs more supervision after bowel movements and after meals, and a high fibre diet with plenty of fluids may help;
- incontinence pads are useful only if they are of the correct size and type and the resident is willing to keep them on.
- many male residents find conveens puzzling and a nuisance and pull them off and it may be worth concentrating on regular toileting.

Inappropriate sexual behaviour

This can range from masturbating and stripping off in public, to simply wanting to hold hands with a member of either sex. Views of what constitutes 'sexual' and 'inappropriate' vary. Some staff may find it appalling that two residents should hold hands and constantly kiss and cuddle one another, whilst others may be pleased that the pair are enjoying one another's company.

It is more common for recently bereaved residents and those who are used to an affectionate relationship prior to coming into the home to seek a close

that the rapid deterioration in Mrs Z.'s mental state coincided with an increase in the dose of digoxin. Withdrawing the chlorpromazine and changing to a different cardiac drug produced remarkable results; although still confused Mrs Z. was no longer disturbed, and stopped falling over. She went home after three weeks.

The best principle of medication is to give the smallest effective dose over a restricted period, and only after all alternative methods have failed and the person is distressed or distressing others. Medication should not be the first port of call, and if behavioural techniques are used then they should be given a chance to work. Drugs can be seen as a quick way of doing something definite. Often the immediate carers put pressure on the qualified staff to do something to make the patient more 'manageable'. It has been shown that there is high drug usage in homes where there is poor staff morale, a negative approach to the residents and poor management support.

CARE OF THE RELATIVES

Supporting the family is just as important as caring for the resident. Many relatives are puzzled and distressed by their relative's behaviour; spending time with them explaining what is happening in the brain and therefore the causes of consequent behaviours can help them make sense of what is happening to the sufferer. A search for a meaning is part of the grieving process.

Relatives often need support in helping them to recognize their feelings and to regard them as normal. Some of the many feelings expressed—anger, grief, resentment, guilt, embarrassment, helplessness, hatred and confusion— are all normal reactions associated with bereavement, and some find it difficult to understand why they are reacting like this when the person has not yet died. Our role is to help them understand that they are grieving for the loss of someone they previously knew: 'He is not the same man I married'.

Probably the feeling expressed most often by relatives when a resident comes into a nursing home is one of guilt and helplessness: 'Why can't I care for them?'. One devoted husband felt he had reneged on his marriage vows by bringing his wife to a nursing home: 'I feel as though I've divorced her'. I find it extremely useful to tell relatives that now the confused person is in the home, they may be inclined to express their feelings of guilt in different ways: 'She didn't do that at home', when it was the reason the person was admitted; 'My mum isn't as bad as the others'; 'You don't look after mum like I did'. Sometimes it is very much easier to complain that 'One of mum's cardigans is missing' than to look at a deteriorating person.

As carers we often wrongly assume that all relatives have good relationships with residents. Miss B. appeared very hostile towards all the staff whenever she visited her mother. One day she was asked how she and her mother had got on and she broke down, saying she had never got on with her mother because her mother had been selfish towards the father when he was dying of cancer. After many conversations the woman was able to see that her behaviour to staff resulted from unresolved feelings towards her mother, and she was later able to start to feel that some of her mother's 'bad' behaviour may have been caused by the early stages of Alzheimer's disease.

By giving carers time in an informal setting such as a carers' group pays dividends; and although time consuming, on-going talk which builds trust and confidence will help acceptance of the resident's condition. Some relatives benefit from an analytical approach, others seek only reassurance. We are able to offer the following explanations:

- make your visiting times short, so that residents don't become distressed as a result of over-stimulation;
- remember that letting a resident sleep occasionally in her day clothes rather than forcing her to get undressed is not negligence, it is part of the management of the condition;
- things may go missing because residents are allowed to wander freely without the doors in the living area being locked.

An important aspect to note is that staff often take on the role of the family and need just as much care and supervision. One of the drawbacks of primary care is that staff are very closely involved with residents on a day-to-day basis and sometimes become over-protective. A possessive 'freezing out' of other staff who 'don't understand' may result. Staff have been known to show hostility towards the resident's relatives as they become more and more engrossed in the care and come to see the family as interfering. Staff may well grieve as much as the family when the resident dies.

CONTINUING CARE

As the resident's health deteriorates to the extent that they are not eating and drinking and require constant physical care, it is highly preferable that the resident stays in the care of staff with whom they have built a strong relationship through the primary nursing system. Primary nursing helps the family to cope with the dying relative; they can communicate more effectively with staff they know and trust, since they are better able to express their feelings. As the staff's understanding of the resident and his family builds up, it is wise to discuss the resident's death in advance, however difficult this may be. In an ideal world, all nursing homes would continue care to the end of the resident's days.

CONCLUSION

Undoubtedly, caring for the confused is a demanding and stressful job. Whilst nobody would suggest that a nursing home will ever represent a cure for Alzheimer's disease, a good nursing home will aim to create a worthwhile quality of life. It is certainly a great advantage if the environment is designed for the special needs of the elderly confused, but there is no substitute for a positive and practical approach to care. Seeing residents as individuals and building strong relationships with each of them will create a sense of identity and the feeling amongst residents, relatives and staff alike that time spent in the home is a part of life rather than a prelude to death.

REFERENCES

Argyll, N., Jestice, S. and Brooke, C. (1985). The psycho-geriatric patient: their supporters' problems. *Age Aging,* **14**, 335–360.
Birchmore, T. and Clague, S. (1983). A behavioural approach to reduce shouting. *Nursing Times*, **79**, 37–39.
Henderson, B. (1980). *Forgetting but not Forgotten. Residential Care of Mentally Frail Elderly People*, Uniting Church, Melbourne.

BIBLIOGRAPHY

Alzheimer's Disease Society (1990). *Questions and Answers*. The Alzheimer Disease Society, London.
Forsythe, E. (1990). *Alzheimer's Disease—the Long Bereavement.* Faber and Faber, London.
Jorm, A.F. (1987). *Understanding Senile Dementia.* Croom Helm, London.
Kitwood, T. and Bredin, K. (1991). *Person to Person—a Guide to the Care of Those with Failing Mental Powers.* Bradford Dementia Research Group, University of Bradford.
Riordan, J. and Whitmore, B. (1990). *Living with Dementia.* Manchester University Press.
Stokes, G. (1986). *Shouting and Screaming.* Winslow, Bicester.
Stokes, G. (1986). *Wandering.* Winslow, Bicester.
Stokes, G. (1987). *Aggression.* Winslow, Bicester.
Woods, R.T. (1987). *Alzheimer's Disease—Coping with a Living Death.* Souvenir Press, London.
Woods, R.T. and Britton, P.G. (1985). *Clinical Psychology with the Elderly.* Croom Helm, London.

13

The Social Consequences of Dementia

HARRY CAYTON

Director, Alzheimer's Disease Society, London, UK

INTRODUCTION

Dementias are of course physical illnesses with physical causes. This chapter however concentrates on the social aspects of dementia; the consequences of the identification and diagnosis of Alzheimer's disease or some other dementia and the progress of the disease. I say 'identification and diagnosis' because this is a social act, which makes dementia apparent and which sets in train a series of reactions and events, and is as significant in determining the impact of the disease on the person, the family and on the providers of health and social care as the symptoms of the disease itself.

Alzheimer's disease and other dementias may be seen as pre-eminently social illnesses. They progress by disturbing the relationship between the person and his or her world, affecting and eventually destroying perception, language, cognition and social behaviour. Our memory of who we are, of our surroundings, of people we know, of our own past and our own present, is the essence of our personality. The disintegration of the personality in the person with dementia destroys the complex web of social relationships and social interaction which surrounds us as individuals. Dementia changes the social behaviour and the social environment, not only of the person who has the condition but of their partner, family, friends, and neighbours, and demands the creation of a specialized network of professional care and support.

THE SOCIAL IMPACT ON THE SUFFERER

The social impact of dementia on the person is obvious. People change over time from being autonomous human beings to complete physical and mental

151

dependency. It is the mental deterioration combined with progressive physical dependency which makes dementia socially so disruptive. If a person loses their ability to understand, to speak, to communicate, to reason, then the people surrounding that person must take on new responsibilities, responsibilities which have ethical, legal and financial implications as well as for health and social care.

The person with dementia voluntarily or involuntarily has to give up control of his/her own affairs. Earlier diagnosis of Alzheimer's disease has implications for GPs, social services and perhaps in due course for medical treatment, but it also introduces the opportunity for the person with dementia to make some plans about their own financial and domestic affairs while they still have insight. An Enduring Power of Attorney can only of course be enacted if a person still has comprehension and will. The alternative is the Court of Protection which, however benign its officers, is expensive, cumbersome, restrictive and an added burden on the carer/receiver.

Other ethical and social questions arise in terms of consent to treatment. The Alzheimer's Disease Society welcomes the debate on 'Living Wills' and the possibility of 'Health Proxies' being appointed. As earlier diagnosis comes about through increased awareness and perhaps physiological tests there will be pressure for legal changes to improve this inadequate area of our law.

THE SOCIAL IMPACT ON CARERS

There are an estimated 1.7 million carers in the United Kingdom looking after disabled and/or elderly relatives. Of these some half million are involved in caring for someone with dementia. Half of those are looking after someone over 85 (Cornwall, 1989). There is in fact no evidence to support the often repeated view that families in Britain have given up their caring role.

These carers may be elderly themselves, often the partners of those they care for. The impact of caring extends to every area of their lives. It affects their relations with their children if there are any, with other members of the family, with neighbours, friends and the local community.

In some instances a community may be supportive, in many others people are rejected. The behaviour of people with dementia can be embarrassing or difficult in the street or in shops. They and their partners may be ostracized. The local pub which someone has visited for 20 years may close its doors to them. Friends no longer call. As the disease progresses both the carer and the sufferer become trapped in their own home. The carer's own life becomes entirely circumscribed by the 24 hour task of caring.

The carer's health is also likely to suffer. Stress and physical illness in carers have been well documented by Levin and others (Levin *et al.*, 1989) with consequences for social services and primary health care.

The abuse of elderly vulnerable people has received attention in Britain recently in ways which distort and exaggerate the situation.

Abuse, whether physical, sexual or psychological comes from a breakdown in relationships. As we have seen, in dementia social disturbance is an unavoidable part of the disease. Where abuse arises in caring relationships it may spring from two different sources. First the relationship may always have been damaged, unsatisfactory or abusive. People in such situations should never be required to care. Secondly, the relationship may become abusive because of lack of support for the carer by professional services.

We do need to look more at the prevention of abuse of older dependent people but we must not blame carers who are as much victims of the situation as the person with dementia.

The social impact on younger carers

The social consequences of dementia may be more extreme if the carer is a younger person, most usually a daughter. Within the self selecting group of carers who form the membership of the Alzheimer's Disease Society two-thirds care for a partner and one-third are children caring for a parent. In these situations the financial consequences are often considerable.

A daughter will probably have given up work to care. The loss of income resulting from that is in no way made up by state benefits and allowances. There is a long-term loss of pension contributions and savings and the opportunity for re-employment for ex-carers when parents have died or gone into a nursing home is remote. Such people are often condemned to poverty both as carers and later in their own old age.

This poverty is reinforced by our Government's policy of including houses in the calculation of a person's assets for benefit purposes. A carer may continue to live in their parent's home after the parent has gone into a nursing home but if they want to sell the house to release some capital social services may make a claim on the proceeds of the sale against their parent's residential care costs. This leaves the former carer without home or capital. These problems are particularly acute where the state does not recognize the relationship between carer and the person with dementia.

If the current practice by health authorities of reducing NHS continuing care beds and transferring responsibility for the elderly mentally ill to social services continues, more and more people will have to sell their homes to pay for the cost of their own long-term care. This wealth locked up in property will not pass down to the next generation as the present Prime Minister has said he wants it to. It will pass down to the providers of private nursing care.

The younger sufferer

The financial consequences are even greater for those who develop Alzheimer's disease in mid-life and for their families. Someone who is in their forties loses job and income at a time when perhaps their children are growing up. People with early features of dementia have been sacked before the illness is diagnosed with loss of unemployment and sickness benefit. Partners usually try to work as long as possible but eventually they too have to give up their job to care full-time.

The loss of two wage earners in a family does not only mean poverty and deprivation for them and their children but is a loss to society as a whole. The family has become dependent on the state rather than a contributor to it.

Estimates of numbers of younger people with dementia in Britain are between 14 000 and 17 000 (Alzheimer's Disease Society, 1992). Specific provision for these people and their families by most health authorities and social services is woefully inadequate or non-existent.

CONSEQUENCES FOR THE STATE

Demographic changes

Dementia will be a major health and social care problem for the rest of this century and beyond.

There has been a revolution in health in the developed world during this century. The infectious and contagious diseases which at the beginning of this century were the main cause of death have almost been eliminated. This reduction in disease means that since the 1950s the number of people over 60 in Europe has increased by 160%, while the population as a whole has increased by 31%. The over 85s have increased by 440% in that period.

It is estimated by the World Health Organization that six to eight million people have dementia in Europe.

In Britain predictions by the Alzheimer's Disease Society suggest that the present number of 600 000 people with dementia will grow by approximately 150 000 to 750 000 30 years from now (Table 1). This growth will come about as a direct result of people living longer, an increase in the number of older people and ironically as a result of better and earlier identification and diagnosis (Alzheimer's Disease Society, 1992). The consequences of this for health authorities is clear. Every regional health authority should have an explicit strategic overview of services for people with dementia (Table 2) who represent a significant health need in every area. To date guidance from the NHS Executive on planning for people with dementia has been virtually non-existent. Dementia is mentioned in the 'Health of the Nation' but

Table 1. Predictions for dementia.[a]

Year	Prevalence of dementia				Total population
	40–64	65–79	80+	Total 40+	
1991	14 670	196 280	387 600	598 550	22 743 000
2001	16 049	194 748	449 200	659 997	24 283 000
2011	17 977	198 740	487 200	703 917	26 695 000
2021	17 261	240 480	495 000	752 741	27 129 000

[a]Based on 1989 OPCS figures. Reproduced with permission, from the Alzheimer's Disease Society (1992).

Table 2. Regional health authorities and dementia in the over 65s.[a]

		Over 65 population (1989)	People with dementia
1.	West Midlands	775 000	38 750
2.	Trent	726 000	36 300
3.	SE Thames	630 000	31 500
4.	North West	622 000	31 000
5.	South West	588 000	29 400
6.	NE Thames	578 000	28 900
7.	Yorks	571 000	28 550
8.	Wessex	507 000	25 350
9.	SW Thames	502 000	25 100
10.	NW Thames	500 000	25 000
11.	Northern	480 000	24 000
12.	Wales	476 000	23 800
13.	Mersey	367 000	18 350
14.	E Anglia	342 000	17 100
15.	Oxford	335 000	16 750
16.	N Ireland	194 000	9 700

[a]Reproduced with permission, from Alzheimer's Disease Society (1992), source: *Regional trends 26* (1991) (using 5% prevalence).

no targets or specific action are described by the Government (HMSO, 1992).

It is important however to recognize that this growth in the number of people with dementia is not a tidal wave threatening to overwhelm us. It is a steady growth but it is manageable if we recognize the existence of the problem and plan care and health services. One in four people over 85 may develop dementia, but three in four won't. Negative messages about older people and the negative images frequently used in the press, advertizing and the television must have a negative impact on political will and planning. A recent survey by Age Concern suggested that young people had an almost universally negative view of the horrors of 'growing old'; a view not shared at all by old people themselves (Age Concern, 1992). A positive commitment to quality of life for all older people needs positive recognition of their place in society.

Costs

The annual cost in Britain of caring for people with disabling mental illness, including dementia, has been estimated at £3 billion (Murphy, 1991). It is actually difficult to know if we must anticipate a rapidly rising cost or if other factors will come into play. Estimates of the numbers of people with dementia are insufficient in themselves, as uncertainty about further levels of health and social care or about the impact of changing social patterns or of possible treatments in the future all contribute to a complex equation.

There is considerable disagreement too about the real impact of an ageing population on health. It is not axiomatic that as life expectancy increases, morbidity will increase and the cost of health and social care will rise. The 'compression of morbidity' hypothesis presumes that as life expectancy increases the onset of chronic illness is prevented or delayed so that the morbidity reduces and costs are also compressed (Keen, 1992).

Reality will probably lie somewhere between the two positions. Although improvements in health, including control of blood pressure and strokes, should reduce multi-infarct dementias for instance, AIDS related dementia is likely to increase.

Earlier and better diagnosis will also increase the demand for services and if drug treatments do become available the involvement of GPs and other medical professionals in care will increase.

THE SOCIAL IMPACT OF TREATMENT

There will of course be drugs in the next few years which have an effect on the symptoms of dementia. I cannot agree at this time with those who see drug treatments as being likely to have a dramatic impact on either people with dementia or on the way we care. Their impact will be gradual, only certain patients will be able to benefit, the cost will limit universality and availability and they will present new ethical dilemmas. A drug which improves memory and cognition may not necessarily improve quality of life as perceived by the person with dementia, and if drugs delay but do not reverse decline carers may face even more years of distressing and exhausting responsibility.

This is not to say, of course, that work on drugs should not continue but the social nature of Alzheimer's disease means that many factors affect drug trials and their outcome. Patients may improve because they are given attention and their carers are highly motivated during a trial. The consequence of successful drug developments go well beyond their effect on the person with dementia alone.

CONCLUSIONS

Care in the community is the basis of the Government's strategy for the chronically disabled. It depends of course on the existence of a community willing to take on that responsibility. Although I have already said that families are continuing to care, there will increasingly be people who have no immediate family. More and more people live alone, families are smaller, divorces are increasing in number, children live further away from their parents. Figures from the Institute of Gerontology (Gerontology Data Service) suggest that while 18.4% of the population over 40 live alone, 31.4% of disabled people are in that position.

It is because dementia is so much a social illness; so interwoven with the way we organize our society and care within it, and so sensitive therefore to changes in society that it is difficult to predict the long-term impact of the different elements in the equation.

It is apparent that the social consequences of dementia are many and varied. The illness starts by affecting the social relations, the legal and financial autonomy of the individual, as it progresses its influence extends to partner, family and the community. Social services will need to put enormous resource into support for people with dementia and their carers if community care is to work. Health services will become increasingly involved as earlier diagnosis and identification become more frequent and as drug treatments become available.

A growing number of older people in society will require a redirection of resources towards their priorities and their needs. Changing patterns of family life will also impact on the way in which care is organized and the financial consequences of paying for care through taxes, health insurance or the savings and capital of elderly people themselves will extend from one generation to the next.

The experience of dementia for the person who suffers from it is of disorientation, confusion, loss and isolation. It is particularly ironic that as the person with dementia feels and becomes less and less part of society, of the physical and human world around them so society needs to become more and more deeply engaged with their life.

In 1623 John Donne, the poet and Divine, was seriously ill with a prolonged and nearly fatal illness. He wrote a series of meditations on sickness and dying, '*Devotions on Emergent Occasions*'. One much quoted, and misquoted, passage is particularly appropriate to the social illness of dementia and the engagement of the individual and society which it embodies.

No man is an Iland, intire of it self;
every man is a peece of the Continent,
a part of the maine; if a clod bee washed
away by the Sea, Europe is the lesse,
as well as if a mannor of thy friends
or of thine owne were; any mans
death diminishes me, because I am involved in
mankinde; And therefore
never send to know for whom the
bell tolls; it tolls for Thee.

(John Donne, 'Devotions XVII', 1624.)

The ageing population of Europe is not 'them'; it is us.

REFERENCES

Age Concern (1992). *Dependency: The Ultimate Fear.* Age Concern, London.

Alzheimer's Disease Society (1992). *The Alzheimer's Report: Caring for Dementia: Today and Tomorrow.* Alzheimer's Disease Society, London.

Cornwall, J. (1989). *The Consumer's View: Elderly People and Community Health Services.* King's Fund Centre, London.

HMSO (1992). *The Health of the Nation: A Strategy for Health in England.* HMSO Books, Norwich.

Keen, J. (1992). *Dementia.* Office of Health Economics, London.

Levin, E., Sinclair, I. and Gorbach, P. (1989). *Families, Services and Confusion in Old Age.* Gower, Aldershot.

Murphy, E. (1991). *After the Asylums, Community Care for People with Mental Illness.* Faber & Faber, London.

V

Current Research and Prospects for New Treatment Strategies

The Management of Alzheimer's Disease
Edited by Gordon K. Wilcock
©1993 Wrightson Biomedical Publishing Ltd

14

Problems of Clinical Research in Dementia

ANTHONY CLARKE

Associated Director (Europe), Besselaar, Maidenhead, UK

CLASSICAL DRUG DEVELOPMENT TRIALS

The classical approach to investigating the effects of a new medication requires a randomized, placebo-controlled, double-blind, parallel group clinical trial; often with a third treatment arm using a standard reference drug. This allows for the assessment of absolute efficacy, as demonstrated by superiority over placebo, and of relative efficacy compared with the reference. In terms of drug safety, the excess of adverse events observed over the placebo rate helps to identify drug-related events as opposed to disease-related events. The comparison of the quantitative and qualitative adverse event profiles against the reference, gives an indication of whether the new drug is likely to represent an advance in terms of acute drug toxicity and tolerability (for general discussion see Colton, 1974). In order to control for confounding variables, such trials frequently have tight entry criteria that define the patient population strictly, and as such can restrict severely the entry of patients with concurrent diseases and those receiving concomitant medication. This leads to most trials being conducted in predominantly young, otherwise healthy patients who do not suffer from multiple pathology and who do not require multiple drug therapy. Such patients can also give reliable written informed consent, which is a requirement for trials conducted according to European Community or Food and Drug Administration Good Clinical Practice.

For diseases with easily recognizable signs and symptoms and with objective measures of efficacy, this approach is defendable on strong scientific and methodological grounds. For example, for patients with mild to moderate hypertension, the principal signs are not disputed, and blood pressure provides an objective measure of drug efficacy. This allows the use of unequivocal diagnostic entry criteria and of strong clear-cut efficacy endpoints to determine success of clinical outcome. It also allows the calculation of sample sizes to be performed with a high degree of confidence, since the expected treatment difference and the inter-patient variability of blood pressure are readily quantifiable. Since the scientific integrity of the entire trial design rests upon the ability of the trial to detect treatment differences if they exist, the ability to estimate accurately the expected efficacy differences and the variability of the test measures, is central to the whole approach to trial design.

Despite the lack of biological markers, of objective diagnostic procedures and of outcome measures, many trials in psychiatric disorders can follow the general approach outlined above. For example, the core symptomatology in major depression is generally agreed and recognizable. Diagnostic criteria such as the DSM-IIIR (American Psychiatric Association, 1987), although not beyond dispute on fine detail, can provide the basis for agreed trial diagnostic entry criteria. Furthermore, validated and sensitive test instruments such as the Hamilton Rating Scale for Depression (HAMD; Hamilton, 1960) or Montgomery–Åsberg Depression Rating Scale (MADRS; Montgomery and Åsberg, 1979), provide reliable subjective substitutes for objective measures of outcome.

The development of the HAMD and MADRS required two prerequisites: recognition of the core symptomatology, and the existence of antidepressant drugs with which to test and refine the developing scales. This led to a self-perpetuating circle: drugs with antidepressant activity helped to validate the scales and the scales helped to detect the effects of newer drugs.

DRUG TRIALS IN SENILE DEMENTIA

For drug trials in senile dementia, we are much further back on the road to the development of sensitive scales and of effective drugs. The patients to be studied are by definition old. Consequently, we ought to expect that these patients will share the characteristics of other non-dementing elderly people, including frailty, fear, infirmity, and depression (see review by Pitt, 1982). Indeed, some of these characteristics may well be exaggerated in a dementing patient and may also be accompanied by other features such as confusion, disorientation, agitation and aggression. All of these characteristics contribute to the clinical and logistic difficulties of conducting dementia trials.

Similarly, the elderly as a whole may receive several drugs for the various diseases often associated with advancing age. Patients commonly present who are taking antihypertensive agents, hypnotics, anti-arthritis drugs and so on. This is often not taken into consideration in the design of many dementia trials, where elderly dementing, but otherwise healthy patients, are studied.

This creates several problems: these patients are quite rare (they have been termed 'the super-elderly' because they are so atypical), and there can be problems in the interpretation of the results of such trials as the patients studied are probably not representative of the population of demented patients as a whole.

THE APPROPRIATENESS OF PLACEBO-CONTROLLED TRIALS IN DEMENTIA

So far, no 'gold standard' antidementia drug has emerged. Therefore, the sound ethics of placebo-controlled trials in dementia ought not to be in question. Indeed, even for those patients who may be randomized to receive placebo, the additional investigations they receive may be of benefit to them. For example, diagnostic procedures used to assess the suitability of patients for inclusion in the trial, may reveal previously undiagnosed pathology, which would have remained undiagnosed if it were not for the additional clinical attention the patient received as part of the screening procedures for the trial. Until effective antidementia drugs become available, even an experimental treatment may be seen as the patient's only hope, and can lead to pressures to avoid the use of placebo control groups. However, without the placebo control the degree of improvement seen in treated patients cannot be put into true perspective, and as such will remain a relatively anecdotal result. Consequently, rather than advancing our knowledge of dementia and its treatment, such uncontrolled studies merely add to our lack of knowledge and represent a lost opportunity.

It is common for patients enrolled into short-term placebo-controlled clinical trials to be allowed to enter a longer-term treatment protocol. Consequently, the use of placebo in these circumstances does not represent a denial of treatment, but a delay of treatment. A delay of treatment of a few months, within the timecourse of deterioration associated with dementia, is not unreasonable in most cases. Furthermore, should the longer-term protocol continue with blinded medication, it is possible that some patients may be treated with placebo in the longer term (assuming that the investigating physician has determined that their continued participation in the trial is acceptable). This gives the additional advantage that long-, as well as short-term comparative measures of efficacy and safety against placebo can be made. This may be particularly important, since antidementia drugs once marketed will be used clinically in the long term, and their long-term safety and efficacy profile should be determined. As well as providing short-term improvement in cognition, a drug may also slow the rate of deterioration of cognitive function. In the absence of longer-term placebo-controlled data, this lack of deterioration may be more difficult to detect.

Finally, it is well recognized that many demented patients treated with placebo are capable of showing an improvement in cognitive function, although the effect is relatively short-lived. The inclusion of a placebo treatment arm to a trial protocol allows the timecourse of this placebo effect to be quantified, and for the true drug response above and beyond it to be recognized.

DIAGNOSTIC STANDARDS

All clinical trials need a clear definition of the disease under study. For dementia, this should be in the form of an accepted disease entity with recognizable pathology and indicative symptoms, such as senile dementia of the Alzheimer type (SDAT) or multi-infarct dementia (MID), and not a vague description of diffuse symptomatology such as cerebrovascular insufficiency. The degree of agreement on the acceptability of the DSM-IIIR dementia definitions is not so high as for other diagnoses. Nonetheless, there is great strength in using published research criteria as a way of ensuring that the patient population studied is recognizable by other research groups. This approach also helps in the process of reaching consensus on the degree to which results can be generalized to other patients.

DISEASE PROGRESSION AND SEVERITY

Primary dementias are progressive diseases. Consequently there can be two possible aims of treatment: to produce improvement in symptoms, and/or to attenuate the rate of deterioration. It is important to distinguish between these at the trial design stage. It is clear that chances of demonstrating *major* improvements in patients with advanced and severe disease are slim, due to the extent of neurone loss that has already taken place. This suggests therefore that the research effort should be concentrated on patients with mild to moderate disease. In such patients, the capacity to improve (or the possibility of slowing the deterioration) is greater, and hence the odds of a successful outcome from the trial are more favourable. The definition of mild to moderate is often made in terms of the score achieved on the trial's primary efficacy rating scale, such as the Alzheimer's Disease Assessment Scale (Rosen *et al.*, 1984) or Mini-Mental Scale (Folstein *et al.*, 1975).

A problem arises however, that since patients with milder disease are earlier in their timecourse of the disease, the diagnosis is less certain. For example, for a newly diagnosed patient, consideration should be given to the possibility of identifiable causes for the patient's symptoms (this will be discussed later). Until an attempt to do so has been made, a diagnosis of early (mild) dementia has to be considered to be an uncertain diagnosis, although some work has been performed to try to reduce this uncertainty (for example, see Copeland *et al.*, 1986).

LOCATION OF PATIENTS

In general terms, patients with advanced dementia become hospitalized since the degree of care they require becomes increasingly difficult to provide in the community. Conversely, the milder patients are most unlikely to be found in hospital. This presents a problem for therapeutic trials: the staff and facilities required to conduct research on demented patients are found mostly in hospital centres and not in the community. However, there are a number of ways in which this problem can be overcome. First, established specialist dementia research centres and physicians with an interest in dementia research are generally known to local general practitioners (GPs) by reputation, and it is likely that with a little effort, these GPs can be persuaded to refer their patients earlier rather than later. Secondly, there are a number of established memory clinics in the UK and elsewhere (for example, see Van der Cammen *et al.*, 1987), where a good liaison between the hospital and community physicians has led to the rapid referral of mild to moderate cases to the hospital-based research clinic. This arrangement has beneficial effects all round; the patient receives better investigation, the GP does not have to attempt to treat a patient with an (as yet) largely untreatable disease and the hospital research group receives patients who are appropriate for research purposes. Finally, a development in recent years has been to perform trials directly in general practice. This requires a great deal of careful training and support for GPs, but removes the burden of frequent hospital visits for the patient, and leaves them treated at home in familiar surroundings by their local doctor who is known to them.

There are a number of measures that can be employed to ensure that the GP receives adequate support before and during the trial. Dementia is a disease dealt with more frequently by psychiatrists, geriatricians and neurologists than by GPs. The help and advice of a local 'expert' such as a psychiatrist or neurologist for each GP, can be helpful. This help could be in the form of discussing the diagnosis for a particular case, of a second opinion or of the interpretation of items on rating scales for a particular patient. The local 'expert' can also help in training groups of GPs and their support staff such as practice nurses and health visitors. This last point is very important: the management of dementia often requires a multidisciplinary approach— dementia trials always need a multidisciplinary approach.

Even in general practice, the flow of suitable patients may be low and the access to hospital expertise and facilities difficult to obtain. There are a number of methods that GPs can use in order to facilitate the recognition of potential patients. All need careful and tactful handling, but if used appropriately can be valuable. All patients of the appropriate age range may be actively screened with a simple test to detect early memory loss. The concept of active screening is accepted and widely used for physical illness, such as hypertension or diabetes, so why not for early dementia? Posters in waiting rooms can increase awareness of memory loss both in patients and their relatives, who can be encouraged to inform the doctor if they think that they or a member of their family may be affected. Finally, as part of an on-going 'well elderly' clinic, potential patients can be contacted and invited to attend the surgery for a simple test of cognitive function, along with the more common batteries of diagnostic tests for the other diseases commonly found in the elderly.

These approaches help to identify potential candidates for inclusion in a trial as early in the course of disease progression as possible, but also increase the chances of misdiagnosis: newly diagnosed patients do not have an established history of disease progression to help support the diagnosis.

PATIENT POPULATION ENRICHMENT

The term patient population enrichment refers to any process by which the pool of patients with a *potential* diagnosis of dementia is reduced to one where the diagnosis is more certain. Consequently the chances of observing a favourable drug response to an effective drug are increased. This increased confidence of the certainty of the diagnosis should help to reduce the inter-patient variability in response rates, since patients with an antidementia drug who do not suffer from the disease are less likely to show improvement in the medium term than those who do. Assuming the drug has true antidementia activity, and not a generalized action on for example mood, attention or motivation, it is likely that only patients with established cognitive impairment will respond.

The following two methods of patient population enrichment are by no means mutually exclusive, and their use would depend on the aim of the trial being performed.

Therapeutic enrichment by treatment response

For trials where improvement is likely in the short term, for example within three months, the population can be enriched using response to the study drug itself. In this trial design, all patients receive active drug therapy in the

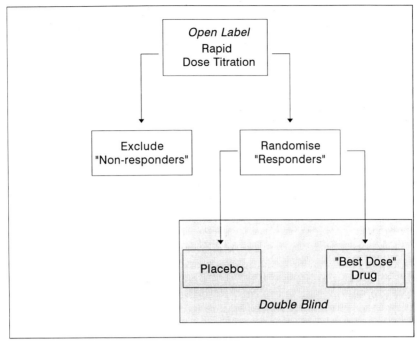

Figure 1. An example of a therapeutic enrichment trial design. All patients are treated with increasing dosages of the trial drug, typically for about 1–3 months. Patients not showing a response ('non-responders') are excluded. The remainder ('responders') are randomized to the 3–6 month double-blind phase, where they receive either placebo or trial drug given at their 'best dose' from the open label phase.

short term, using a rapid dose titration. The purpose is to try to identify as quickly as possible those patients who show a positive therapeutic response to the drug. Non-responders are excluded from the trial at the end of the short-term dose titration phase. The remainder ('responders') are then randomized to be treated further in the double-blind phase of the trial with either active drug (given at the 'best dose' identified from the short-term titration phase) or with placebo (see Fig. 1). This method ensures that the population studied is *capable* of showing a response; the double-blind phase results demonstrate the *extent* of that response. An example of a trial using this method of enrichment was described by Murphy *et al.* (1991).

There is the potential for ethical concern over this method of enrichment, since patients with a largely untreatable disease are identified, successfully treated for a short time, then (in the placebo group) deliberately denied treatment. The broader ethical view however reveals that if patients were not entered into the trial, they would be untreated anyway. Also, once the relatively short double-blind phase is over, all patients could be transferred to compassionate use of active medication. This method has also been criticized since the population treated consists by definition of 'responders'. Thus the demonstration of drug efficacy in such a population is hardly a surprise. There is also little scope for generalizing the results of the trial to the population of demented patients as a whole. Both criticisms would be entirely justified in a clinical field where there were already in existence a number of active drugs available to treat the disease, or where failure to treat (or deliberately withholding treatment) may be seriously injurious to the patient. Neither of these is true in dementia, where there are no drugs with acceptable clinical utility in widespread use and where the long timescale of patient deterioration means that withholding therapy for a relatively short time is unlikely to lead to any significant long-term negative consequences for the patient.

This method of enrichment is unsuitable for drugs that do not have a rapid onset of action, as the titration phase would have to become unworkably long. There can also be logistic problems in the provision of double-blind medication at the 'best dose'. This can be overcome by choosing a fixed dose for patients randomized to active treatment in the double-blind phase, although the decision as to which dose may not necessarily be an easy one. It should be recognized that dementia is a long-term diagnosis, and a relatively short delay in the provision of blinded medication at 'best dose' may not compromize the trial unreasonably.

Methodological enrichment by exclusion of secondary dementias

It may seem obvious, but by identifying causes for a patient's cognitive impairment, the pool of patients can be reduced by a process of elimination to those with primary dementias. This is not easy to achieve, and the financial and logistic costs are high. This process has been variously described in terms of the reliability of diagnosis of dementia (Homer et al., 1988; O'Connor et al., 1988) and of the 'reversibility' of dementia (Barry and Moskowitz, 1988; Byrne, 1987; Cummings, 1985), but equally applies to the conduct of clinical trials. Table 1 shows a list of some causes of cognitive impairment, and Table 2 shows some of the diagnostic aids to their detection (for detailed discussion see Pearce et al., 1988). It is clear that some diagnoses such as infection may be easier to detect than others. The list of assessments is long, but well researched (McKhann et al., 1984; Wilcock et al., 1989).

The case notes for elderly patients are often inaccurate and incomplete. Thus the notes cannot be relied upon as the only source of historical information about the patient, and may need to be supplemented by other

Table 1. Causes of secondary dementias.

Trauma
    Head injury
    Sub-dural haematoma

Infections
    Brain abscess
    Meningitis/encephalitis
    Neurosyphilis
    Creutzfeldt–Jacob disease

Anoxia
    Hypoconfusional states

Deficiency states
    Vitamin B_{12}, folic acid
    Wernicke–Korsakov's syndrome (thiamine)
    Pellagra

Vascular
    Multi-infarcts
    Binswanger's encephalopathy

Intoxication
    Barbiturates
    Alcoholism
    Amphetamines, Hallucinogens
    Organic poisons, solvents, glue sniffing

Metabolic
    Hypothyroidism
    Hypopituitarism
    Renal failure, dialysis dementia
    Hepatic encephalopathy

Dynamic
    Hydrocephalus

Neoplasms
    Carcinoma or lymphoma

Table 2. Secondary dementia investigation.

Investigation	Results
Blood count	Anaemia
ESR	Connective tissue disorders
Chest X-ray	Bronchial neoplasm, cardiac lesions
Liver function tests	Hepatic failure
VDRL	Neurosyphilis
Serum B_{12}	Vitamin B_{12} deficiency
Red blood cell folate	Folate deficiency
Serum T_3, T_4, TSH	Hypothyroidism
Skull X-ray	Space occupying lesion
CSF	Chronic meningitis or neurosyphilis
EEG	Slowing in primary cerebral atrophies; focal change in space-occupying lesion
ECG	Arrhythmias, ischaemic heart disease, embolism
Angiography	Carotid and cerebral vascular stenoses, occlusions, sub-dural haematoma, tumours
CT or MRI	Central and cortical atrophy, other focal lesions, infarcts, tumours, haematomas

measures such as additional history taking from the patient, and interviews with close relatives.

There may also be problems of interpretation of conflicting results from the battery of diagnostic tests undertaken. For example, in differentiating between SDAT and MID there may be neurological signs indicating focal deficits, but no evidence of infarcts on a CT scan. This may be because the patient has neurological problems largely unrelated to their dementia or because the infarcts were too small to be visualized. Issues such as these need careful consideration at the trial planning stage, and may need occasional review by an independent steering committee during the trial, in order to dictate policy on how to deal with them.

It could be argued that this is not worth the effort or the cost. However some of the dementias found may be reversible and other diagnoses found

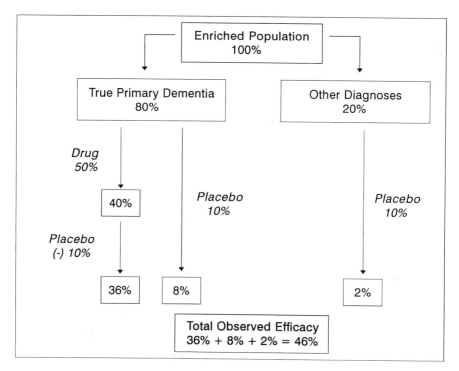

Figure 2. The effect of methodological enrichment on observed therapeutic response. In this theoretical example, the population has been enriched so that 80% of the patients have a true primary dementia and the remainder some other (unknown) diagnosis. If the drug produces a theoretical response in 50% of patients with a true primary dementia, and placebo produces a response in 10% of all patients, the *overall* observed response will be 46%.

The Management of Alzheimer's Disease
Edited by Gordon K. Wilcock
©1993 Wrightson Biomedical Publishing Ltd

15

Alzheimer's Disease and the Pharmaceutical Industry: Resources and Hope

PETER D. STONIER

Medical Director, Hoechst UK Ltd, Hounslow, and Visiting Professor in Pharmaceutical Medicine, HPRU, University of Surrey, Guildford, UK

INTRODUCTION

The medical and social approaches to the management of Alzheimer's disease include the search for medicines which may alleviate the symptoms, halt the progress and even reverse the process of this devastating and mortal disease. Since in today's medical economic climate every effort is being made to contain health care costs, it is pertinent to be reminded that the introduction of new chemical entities, for example medical treatments for chronic diseases including Alzheimer's disease, must be viewed not only through the eyes of researchers hoping for a breakthrough but also through the eyes of those who balance the investment of the health care resources of manpower, time, and money in one area of hopeful endeavour against another.

Alzheimer's disease represents a particularly acute example of the potential conflicts between the allocation of research resources and the increasing hope of a therapeutic breakthrough after a number of exciting leads in the pathophysiology of the disease have suggested routes for therapy. This is because there is currently no effective treatment available for this disease, which afflicts an increasingly ageing population, and yet available health care resources for the sector of the population are forever stretched as increased morbidity takes its toll.

A question is always asked about the purpose of pharmaceutical intervention in a chronic disease of insidious onset which is often well-advanced when diagnosed, particularly when set against the possibilities for effective management of other diseases and afflictions of the elderly. Whilst the answer lies inevitably in the philosophy of a society's approach to the value of individual lives, the impetus to medical research derives from a traditional recognition that palliation based on intervention in a rational pathophysiological model is justified by being at least the first rung on the ladder of disease modification and cure.

PHARMACEUTICAL RESEARCH RESOURCES

The international research-based pharmaceutical industry has been a highly successful product of modern applied science over some four decades and has contributed significantly to the improved health of mankind. It is also a profitable industry and regarded by the stock market as a good area for investment. For countries like the UK it has provided a positive trade balance over many years, and in times of recession provides a beacon of hope for industrial regeneration.

Investment in R&D by the world's pharmaceutical companies had increased to an estimated \$24 billion (revenue and capital) in 1990 (Halliday *et al.*, 1992), with an average annual growth of 16% since 1981 in the major countries, and represents a massive high-risk research effort which is aimed at the discovery and development of new treatments for a wide range of diseases in which central nervous system disorders including Alzheimer's disease feature high on the list. Almost half of the revenue R&D expenditure (46%) in 1989 was allocated in Europe, with 36% in the USA and 15% in Japan.

Three quarters of worldwide revenue expenditure in 1989 was spent on new chemical entities, with discovery research and clinical evaluation each accounting for approximately 30%.

This level of spending on research represents a real increase in that globally there has been a rise in the proportion of R&D revenue expenditure to sales from about 10% in 1981 to 14.6% in 1990.

No proven effective medicine has yet been introduced for Alzheimer's disease, although it has been predicted that products will be introduced within the next few years (Iversen, 1992). This breakthrough, probably in the first instance in symptomatic treatment, is badly needed as a benchmark for the incremental progress which will surely follow towards more effective treatments with an improved risk to benefit ratio, leading perhaps to the goal of disease-modifying agents early in the next century.

To this end, and despite nearly 12 years of development time at a cost of around \$240 million per new chemical entity introduced onto the market, there are some 67 companies worldwide with 180 compounds under development for Alzheimer's disease, of which around 30 have been identified by the Pharmaceutical Manufacturers Association (US) as potentially useful symptomatic treatment (Moran, 1991).

RESEARCH THREATS AND AN INDUSTRY RESPONSE

At the same time, Governments throughout the world, and particularly in Europe, have also been determined to reduce their heavy commitments to health care relative to other sectors of society and see the 'Medicines Bill' as one politically acceptable way to achieve this. To an extent the industry has itself attracted attention as a consequence of its very success. Occasional excessive promotional practices, a continuous media interest in company activity, and a popular moralist view that pharmaceutical companies are, uniquely, profiting from illness, have made the industry an easy target for its detractors and a focus for politicians to be seen to be doing something to control the high cost of health care.

It is possible to summarize the main resource pressures affecting product development (Fig. 1) and the pharmaceutical industry's response to them to ensure its so far continued success as a profitable research industry (Fig. 2).

The main issues therefore are, first, the need to invest enormous sums of money in research and development to achieve novelty, prove efficacy and safety, and meet stringent international regulatory demands; secondly, the commercial pressures to see a return on investment before the patent life

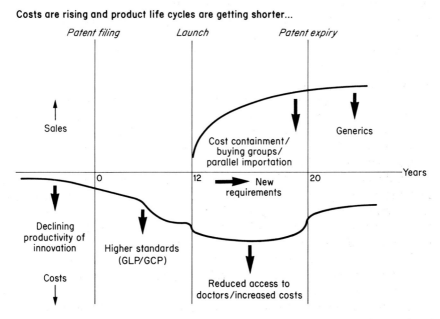

Figure 1. The main resource pressures affecting product development. (Reproduced with permission, © Dr Peter Forrester, Innovex Ltd.)

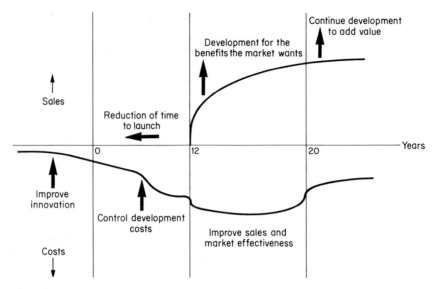

Figure 2. The range of responses from the pharmaceutical industry to the increasing cost of drug development and the reduced product life cycle. (Reproduced with permission, © Dr Peter Forrester, Innovex Ltd.)

expires; and, thirdly, an increasing downward pressure by governments on prices, profit margins, and promotional activity.

R&D expenditure

Because of the increasing difficulties involved in discovery of new chemical entities and the complexity of the processes required to develop a product and bring it successfully to market, $240 million is estimated to be the average investment. This figure relates to all the research to bring a single compound to market, including all the compounds synthesized that do not enter clinical development and also those that commence development but do not successfully reach the market. In a recent survey of 49 leading companies carried out by the Centre of Medicines Research, some companies reported an attrition rate as high as 5200:1 (Halliday *et al.*, 1992). In addition, despite the high spend, the annual total of new chemical entities reaching the world market has declined dramatically from 93 in 1961 to 48 in 1980, even though this was a very innovative period in drug development (Chew *et al.*, 1985). This annual introduction rate now averages around 40.

Despite the apparently large sales figures reported in annual company reports, in fact because of this large R&D expenditure the return to companies is remarkably low. Grabowski (1991) reports a long-term study on the returns to US companies following new drug introductions and found that while net cash flows following launch are high, the return is in fact only between 10–11% which is the same as the opportunity cost of capital. This results in a break-even time averaging 16–17 years for compounds introduced between 1980 and 1984.

Despite these adverse economic trends, in the UK's research environment R&D expenditure on CNS disorders is now second only to cardiovascular disease after significant increases since 1983. The UK industry's R&D spend is currently £1.2 billion, and is the major contributor to all medical research in the country.

Effective patent life

On the issue of patent life, compounds are usually patented as they enter pharmaceutical development. Because the time taken for a successful compound to obtain a Product Licence, remaining patent life has been eroding over many years and is now reduced to anything from 6–13 years.

In 1982 effective patent life based on 438 new chemical entities was estimated by Walker and Prentis (1985) to be as low as 4.7 years for products introduced into the United Kingdom. Since 1984 there have been various schemes to extend effective patent life, resulting in the recent Supplementary Patent Certificate in Europe and, in the US, the Drug Price Competition and Patent Term Restoration Act of 1984, since when the effective patent life of products has averaged about 10 years (Grabowski, 1991).

Despite some promise of a respite in the patent life issue, there is still urgency generated in companies to maximize their return whilst effective patent protection exists and competitors are few. This obviously results in aggressive promotion which also requires huge expenditure and this further reduces the net profit accruing to companies.

Other measures to increase effective patent life must also be considered, such as more efficient and harmonized international development processes and thus reduced times to prepare international dossiers and increased chances of rapid registration in major markets. This is one major expectation of Good Clinical Practice guidance and the Standard Operating Procedures that companies have introduced to harmonize data gathering procedures and validate the resulting data.

For these increased efficiencies in the conduct of research to have any meaning, it is important that results are actually achieved in registration and that new products reach the market as a result of more relevant and high quality data. In this regard and despite exhaustive clinical trials and all the attendant quality and efficiency issues, it is important to recognize the limitations of a preregistration clinical trials programme to produce data on global efficacy or safety of a product. This applies particularly to products for

Table 1. Deficiencies in product
knowledge at the time of licensing.

1. Relative safety and efficacy

2. Individual response
   • Age
   • Co-morbid states

3. Limited clinical data
   • Rare, serious side effects
   • Overdosage
   • Drug abuse potential
   • Teratogenic and carcinogenic effects

4. Drug–drug interactions

5. Drug utilization data

chronic diseases such as Alzheimer's disease and rheumatoid arthritis with insidious onset and course, unknown aetiology and multiple pathology, in which there are difficulties defining diagnostic criteria and clinically relevant drug-sensitive outcome measures.

Rawlins and Jefferys (1991) showed that the mean number of patients treated prior to the grant of a product licence for a new chemical entity was 1480 (range 129–9400).

Table 1 shows some of the deficiencies in knowledge about a product at the time of licence, due to limitation on numbers in clinical trials but also to other factors such as homogeneity of trial population, limitation of dose and duration of treatment, and exclusion of certain patients such as those with concurrent illness or organ failure.

With the awareness of this limited database for new medicines, strategies have been and continue to be developed to monitor drugs carefully once they are marketed and to explore further their properties in terms of efficacy, safety and overall clinical usefulness in patients with the target disease, as well as to extend the knowledge base in respect of pharmacology, mode of action and new indications.

Containing health care costs

At a different level in the therapeutic process, every country with a national health insurance or health service is concerned to contain the costs of medical care. The national medicines bill has received special attention with the introduction in most European countries of price restrictions and negative or limited lists as well as hospital formularies all designed to achieve a lower cost of drugs. This tendency will continue in spite of the protestations of the pharmaceutical industry which has demonstrated repeatedly that relative to a total health care spending, medication costs have remained constant.

In the UK, due to the reorganization of the NHS with increased screening, particularly of the elderly, there is an apparent rise in the drug bill. The recent extension of the selected list of reimbursed medicines in the UK (the Limited List) is further evidence of a continued programme of cost reduction by the government, which the industry believes will seriously undermine its capacity to conduct effective research.

There is also the up-coming problem of pharmaceutical pricing within Europe, which must be resolved in favour of medium to high priced countries in order to protect R&D. So action by governments further reduces profit margins and thus research potential, and while companies still have to promote their products aggressively to achieve a return on investment and satisfy their shareholders, it has led them to search for more acceptable means of doing this and great efforts to improve their image, so that they will not be a political 'soft option' in the future. Companies therefore have responded by putting a greater strategic emphasis on developing compounds in therapeutic areas where there is not a satisfactory treatment available, and where market penetration is achievable not so much by company promotion as by a medically driven perception of real need.

Strategic areas of research include oncological agents, antiviral compounds (especially HIV) and of course chronic degenerative conditions, such as Alzheimer's disease and rheumatoid arthritis. It is in these areas that companies consider the possibility of high return to be greatest, with a lower cost of entry if successful. These strategic decisions and the resultant activities by companies therefore should be viewed not as they traditionally are by detractors as the industry profiting from the chronic misfortunes of society, but as an adaptable research-based ethical industry once more challenging the frontiers of therapeutics in the face of growing economic pressures to curtail this activity. This is well illustrated by the industry's activities in the area of Alzheimer's disease research, where there is clearly a need for greater understanding of the disease and possibilities for therapeutic intervention. Because of the lack of effective therapeutic agents at present, many companies are involved at the forefront of research in this condition. This involves research on the basic pathological mechanisms as well as developing agents based on current knowledge, for example in the area of neurotransmitter deficiency.

Pharmaceutical industry research teams have also made major discoveries in the basic research programmes. For example, a company has cloned the gene coding for a new glutamate receptor which controls the intracellular calcium release within nerve tissue. This could result in drugs being developed to control glutamate which affects processes such as learning and memory.

A monoclonal antibody diagnostic test, which detects a protein marker in cerebral spinal fluid of Alzheimer's patients, has been produced as a result of research into Alzheimer's associated proteins in the brain. This assay incorporates the monoclonal antibody into an enzyme-linked sandwich immunoassay and it may well be that this may prove helpful for early diagnosis in the future.

Such programmes can only be undertaken because of the large resources of the industry but it is increasingly being realized by companies that one of the most promising ways forward is by collaboration with basic research workers at universities and other institutions. Both industry and academia seek collaborative programmes of research and major investments have been made by companies such as SmithKline Beecham in Oxford, Astra at the Institute of Neurology and Parke-Davis in Cambridge.

There is also more direct support of clinical investigations in the field as the industry tests its compounds on patients. This collaboration results in improved diagnostic procedures, more sophisticated clinical trial designs and a positive interchange of ideas and techniques. The money coming into clinical departments also has a spin-off in providing funds for other research areas.

Both academia and industry have recognized the need to pool resources for effective developments of medicines, and in the coming years there is bound to be more collaboration between academia and industry as well as between companies within the pharmaceutical industry itself.

Finally, companies are gradually realizing that they have a real part to play in medical education. They are therefore increasing their contributions to true scientific meetings and exchange of information, both pre- and post-marketing, and also producing more scientifically relevant literature and information. This educational effort by companies greatly assists the flow of information between workers in the field and also keeps medical practitioners informed and therefore abreast of current trends and advances in treatment.

On the resource issue therefore, whilst the threats are there, the industry is at present still a thriving concern, albeit with fewer larger companies at the forefront of research, but with an undiminished impetus to make breakthroughs in many of the unconquered diseases of which Alzheimer's disease is but one. The industry is focusing its efforts on the needs of its 'customers' in medicine with increasingly interactive and collaborative programmes of research and development, aiming at high quality and efficiency enabling strategic decisions to be made in a timely fashion on the basis of relevant data.

Nevertheless, recent ABPI commentary suggests that, due to the decline in government funding of the UK science base and the consequent shortfall of qualified, skilled staff needed to service the industry's high technology

R&D needs, there is already an unsustainable level of R&D spend, workforce size and inter-dependence between the industry and academic institutes, leading ultimately to a reduction in innovative research (ABPI, 1992).

RESEARCH HOPES IN ALZHEIMER'S DISEASE

There are real expectations for a breakthrough in the treatment of Alzheimer's disease in the next few years, and it would appear that the industry is engaged in three competitive races; first to be the first onto the market with an effective product to treat the symptoms of Alzheimer's disease; secondly to produce and prove real and sustained clinical benefit for Alzheimer's patients and their carers leading ultimately to the introduction of disease-modifying agents; and thirdly to achieve all this before major shifts in the economic trends governing pharmaceutical investment, particularly in R&D, serve to force a strategic rethink on research in these difficult areas of chronic disease.

At present there are no winners in these races, and so there is a unique chance to consider how the current medical model for Alzheimer's disease might change with the introduction of the first effective medicines.

Undoubtedly, the introduction of the first medicines will act as a catalyst for the more effective focusing of resources in research and also in many aspects of the current medical and social approaches to managing the condition.

On the medical side, since there is no effective treatment, there is a tendency to under-diagnose dementia, especially Alzheimer's disease, and to see patients only for associated problems. In the community there is a constant realization of the growing problems of dementia and the limited resources to meet them. The introduction of a medicine would at least help to resolve some of the problems of perception about the incidence, prevalence and course of the disease and to bring a rational scientifically based medical model within the range of physicians, both in the community and in hospital practice.

Diagnostic criteria and differential diagnosis

The availability of a medicine which may be of general benefit to a majority of patients with Alzheimer's disease and of specific, dramatic, benefit to a few would mean that doctors would be encouraged to identify and select those patients who might so benefit, and/or certainly should be offered a closely monitored and supervised therapeutic trial.

It remains to be seen what might become the operational standards of diagnosis in practice, especially general practice; might these be based on clinical trial entry criteria, or European guidelines or a standardized protocol introduced, for instance, by the National Health Service in the UK? Would these include DSM-IIIR criteria, NINCDS/ADRDS criteria, a clinical checklist, or a combination of two or more? Almost certainly a clinical diagnosis of dementia would have to be followed by a differential diagnosis to exclude non-Alzheimer's cases, and this would include a battery of laboratory and clinical tests; but what would be the place of the electroencephalogram or computerized tomography in the routine diagnosis of probable Alzheimer's disease?

Disease assessment measures

How will clinical outcomes be measured in practice when effective thera-peutic agents are widespread? Which of the many assessment scales currently familiar only to clinical trialists might prove useful to those doctors and health care professionals charged with measuring the effectiveness and efficiency of pharmaceutical adjuncts to patient management? Will measures of memory, emotions or behaviours become the clinically relevant yardstick, or clinically relevant combinations of all three as in proposed EC guidelines for clinical trials with psychometric measures of cognitive function and clini-cal global impression together with activities of daily living?

Outcome measures

Clinical research programmes have so far hinted that some treatments may slow down disease progression, but none has yet indicated the likely clinical outcome of pharmaceutical intervention in Alzheimer's disease. Will it be to reduce mortality by halting or reversing the primary disease process or by affecting secondary risk factors such as malnutrition, infections and accidents, or will it be to reduce such morbidity and thus improve the quality of life without necessarily prolonging that life? Or will the main effect be on the carer, responding to the renewed hope and a sense of purpose that medical intervention and interest will bring? Many of these questions and others such as an accurate assessment of risk–benefit of the treatment and the overall cost–benefit of therapeutic intervention can only be approached through the continued research on marketed products.

Disease markers

Whilst conventional research into markers for Alzheimer's disease has produced few leads and investment is likely to be modest and even question-able until it is possibly to respond with prophylactic treatment intervention for the positives, research into the human genome or into amyloid protein fragments may provide potential disease markers.

Patient care

The availability of drug therapy, even of small effect and modest benefit would stimulate an overall consideration of patient management and the respective roles of family carers, general practitioner, hospital and social agencies. The concept of shared care between hospital, community services and family perhaps would become more defined as the responsibilities for diagnosis, disease assessment and monitoring of treatment comes more to the fore and plays a greater role in the overall long-term management plan for the patient.

On the clinical side, therefore, the arrival of therapeutic agents on the market would provide a much needed stimulus to the workings of a rational medical model for the diagnosis and treatment of Alzheimer's disease and in so doing would present unprecedented opportunities for research—epidemiological, clinical, pharmacological and social—into this disease of growing importance to ageing nations.

Benchmark for incremental progress

For pharmaceutical medicine, the introduction of the first agents for Alzheimer's disease will provide a true breakthrough.

The first drugs are likely to be palliative medicines, preceding disease modifying agents by years or decades. They are likely to be of modest effect and overall clinical benefit, albeit in an area where every step of progress deserves to be grasped as a hopeful pointer of more to follow. As is almost traditional in pharmaceutical medicine, and particularly psychopharmacology, early drugs are likely to be 'lead' standards, not 'gold' standards, tools to provide an opportunity to make further scientific revelations about the disease and routes to treatment. Such was the case, for instance, in the concomitant development of lithium therapy and understanding of the management of manic-depressive psychosis and its relationship to other affective disorders.

In the case of Alzheimer's disease such drugs would also help to bring the disease into the medical arena, in terms of improving diagnostic and differential diagnostic criteria, in establishing the epidemiology of the condition and the closely related constellation of dementing illnesses, in defining assessment methods and criteria for treatment and treatment monitoring.

Development of assessment methods

Marketed medicines would provide the stimulus for the validation of assessment scales for pivotal international, harmonized, studies for registration of new products. They would stimulate the development of clinical trial methodology and post-marketing surveillance techniques at an international, even global, level. Cultural factors in Alzheimer's disease across countries would also be scrutinized in this programme of clinical research.

Education about Alzheimer's disease

Undoubtedly there is a need for continuing education about Alzheimer's disease at many different levels. The availability of marketed medicines will provide an enormous stimulus to education in this area, catalysing the collaboration between the medical and social approaches to the management of patients.

SUMMARY

It currently takes about 12 years to develop a new medicine at a cost of $240 million. Whilst the pharmaceutical industry has been a successful innovator over the last 40 years, its resource investment base is under threat from several directions—the escalating cost of R&D, pressure on prices, profits and promotion, generic incursion and, now to a lesser extent, attrition of effective patent life.

The industry has reacted by altering its research strategy and directing more of its resources towards novel areas of medical need such as Alzheimer's disease, improving efficiency and quality of its research, endeavouring to reduce development and registration times and by making better use of promotional and sales resources.

While there is no guarantee that this level of resource investment and research effort will be successful or remain sustainable, currently it is providing a competitive environment for development of therapeutic agents for Alzheimer's disease offering hope of imminent availability of at least modestly effective medicines.

While to date no product has been registered, when this occurs it is expected to provide a benchmark with important effects on the medical and social models for the disease, helping to catalyse several areas of collaborative research and strategies for patient diagnosis, assessment and management.

It is expected that marketed medicines will, as in other areas of psychopharmacology, alter the course of future Alzheimer's disease research, particularly that sponsored by the pharmaceutical industry.

REFERENCES

ABPI (1982). *Agenda for Health, Supporting the Science Base* Association of the British Pharmaceutical Industry, London.

Chew, R., Teeling-Smith, G. and Wells, N. (1985). *Pharmaceuticals in Seven Nations.* Office of Health Economics, London.

Grabowski, H. (1991). *Pharmaceutical Research and Development: Returns and Risk.* CMR Annual Lecture, Centre for Medicines Research, London.

Halliday, R.G., Walker, S.R. and Lumley, C.E. (1992). R&D philosophy and management in the world's leading pharmaceutical companies. *J. Pharm. Med.*, **2**, 139–154.

Iversen, L.L. (1992). *Alzheimer's Disease—The Challenge for Drug Discovery.* CMR Annual Lecture, Centre for Medicines Research, London.

Moran, J. (1991). *Alzheimer's Disease; New Therapies and the World Market.* Financial Times Business Information, London.

Rawlins, M.D. and Jefferys, D.B. (1991). Study of United Kingdom product licence applications containing new active substances, 1987–9. *Br. Med. J.*, **302**, 223–225.

Walker, S.R. and Prentice, R.A. (1985). Drug research and pharmaceutical patents. *Pharm. J.*, **214**, 11–13.

16

The Pharmacodynamics of Velnacrine: Results and Conclusions from Clinical Studies in Healthy Subjects and Patients with Alzheimer's Disease

K. SIEGFRIED

Central Clinical Research/Neuroscience, Hoechst AG, and Associate Professor of Human Psychopharmacology and Clinical Neuropsychology, Joh. Wolfg. Goethe University, Frankfurt, Germany

INTRODUCTION

Velnacrine: a potential Alzheimer's disease agent

Velnacrine is a 1,2,3,4-tetrahydro-9-aminoacridine-1-ol maleate which was selected and developed as an anti-Alzheimer's disease (AD) agent. On the biochemical level, the compound acts as a potent cholinesterase inhibitor which prevents a rapid metabolic inactivation of the neurotransmitter acetylcholine. In various pharmacological models in rodents, velnacrine was proven to enhance learning and retention. It was also shown to reverse memory and learning deficits induced either by scopolamine, an anticholinergic (muscarinic blocking) agent, or by lesions of the nucleus basalis magnocellularis (n.b.m.) (Fielding *et al.*, 1989). The n.b.m. in rats is the equivalent of the nucleus basalis of Meynert complex in man that innervates numerous cholinergic pathways which project to various areas of the cortex (e.g. prefrontal, temporal, parietal).

Pharmacokinetic studies in healthy young and elderly men have shown that oral doses of velnacrine were well absorbed. Peak plasma levels are reached within one hour after oral administration, and the elimination half-life is approximately 2–3 hours. Steady-state plasma levels are reached after approximately three days of repeated oral administration. There is a dose-related increase in absorption (AUCs) and the amount of drug excreted.

Peak plasma levels and AUCs are higher and half-life slightly longer in elderly than in young subjects (Puri et al., 1988).

The selection of velnacrine as a potential Alzheimer's disease agent was based on the central cholinergic deficit hypothesis of AD (Davies, 1981; Coyle et al., 1983). In the early 1980s when velnacrine was synthesized, this hypothesis represented 'the most consistent and most extensive neurochemical abnormality yet detected' in patients with AD (Perry, 1987). The following findings obtained by several separate research groups are in support of this hypothesis. Post-mortem studies have shown that there is a markedly reduced activity (up to 90%) of choline acetyltransferase (CAT) in patients with AD relative to age-matched controls (Davies, 1979, 1981; Perry et al., 1977; White et al., 1977). CAT is an enzyme which catalyses the synthesis of acetylcholine in presynaptic nerve terminals (Kuhar, 1976). As a consequence of the reduced CAT activity, there is a central cholinergic deficit in patients with AD. Another strong piece of evidence in support of the cholinergic deficit hypothesis was the finding that the cholinergic abnormalities correlated with both the number of senile plaques in the brains of these patients and the mental test scores on the Blessed Dementia Scale obtained shortly before their death (Perry et al., 1978). Finally, pharmacological studies in young healthy subjects demonstrated the involvement of the cholinergic system in various types of cognitive abilities, in particular memory functions, typically impaired by AD. The administration of scopolamine, a central cholinergic blocking agent, produces an impairment of memory and attentional performance which resembles cognitive deficiencies in AD and is therefore called 'scopolamine dementia' (Drachman and Leavitt, 1974; Huff et al., 1988; Wesnes and Simpson, 1988). On the other hand, physostigmine, a short-acting cholinesterase inhibitor, was found to enhance cognitive functioning (Davis et al., 1976, 1978, 1981; Drachman and Shahakian, 1980; Christie et al., 1981; Thal and Fuld, 1983; Thal et al., 1983; Blackwood and Christie, 1986). However, due to large interindividual variations in bioavailability and its short elimination half-life (approximately 20 min), the cognitive effects of physostigmine cannot be consistently observed and are only mild and short lasting.

The objectives of pharmacodynamic studies and their special problems with antidementia agents

The objectives of the present chapter are to describe and interpret the effects of velnacrine observed in pharmacodynamic studies. The term 'pharmacodynamic effects' refers to drug effects related to a compound's efficacy. Contrary to the concept of efficacy, however, the term 'pharmacodynamic effects' does not necessarily involve the notion of clinical significance; it does, however, not exclude it. Pharmacodynamic studies in human subjects are usually early clinical studies (phase I and phase IIa) which have the following three objectives.

- First, they are supposed to establish whether the effects observed in pharmacological studies in animals can be replicated in man. This task includes dose extrapolation and dose finding, usually also a change in the route of administration and the dosage schedule. In order to achieve these goals, one has to take into account species-specific differences in metabolism and other pharmacokinetic variables.
- Secondly, it is hoped that they will help the prediction of the efficacy of the test compound in the target group of patients for whom the compound is developed.
- Finally, they are expected to elucidate the mechanism of action underlying the compound's efficacy.

Considering these general objectives for pharmacodynamic trials with potential antidementia (or more specifically Alzheimer's disease) agents, one has to face particular difficulties.

Difficulties in the extrapolation from findings in animals to humans

In addition to the usual extrapolation issues in the transition from animal to man, there is a particular problem with the target symptoms of antidementia agents, the cognitive functions and symptoms. The human cognitive system is much more complex than those found in animals, and there are also species-related differences between these systems. Although basic distinctions of relatively separate functional memory subsystems (e.g. short-term memory or working memory, long-term memory) hold true for both humans and more highly developed animals (e.g. mammals), certain subsystems which are typically affected by AD have no real counterpart in animals and therefore cannot be tested in animal models. One example is semantic memory and the language system in man. The extrapolation issue can also be illustrated by another example. Animal studies of learning and memory typically make use of passive avoidance learning models or, generally speaking, of paradigms of classical and operant conditioning learning. In man, classical and operant conditioning represent a subtype of learning or information acquisition processes but the individual conditioning rates do not correlate with performance measures of more complex language-dependent memory abilities which may suggest that the two abilities also represent biologically separate functional systems.

Difficulties in the prediction of efficacy in patients

As long as there are no established antidementia standard compounds, the predictive validity of both preclinical and phase I pharmacodynamic models will remain uncertain. Even if in your healthy subjects the same functions are tested as those which appear to be affected in the target disease there is no certainty as to whether or not the results have a predictive value for patients. A typical example of this kind of problem is the experience with the development of antidepressants: antidepressants usually do not improve mood aspects in healthy young subjects; this is, however, one of their most pronounced effects in depressed patients. Furthermore, the so-called Yerkes–Dodson law would predict that the effects on cognitive performance of a centrally activating compound will depend on the baseline activation level (Broadhurst, 1959). Therefore one would expect that patients whose cognitive impairment is associated with central nervous underactivation would react very differently to such drugs than (normally activated) young healthy subjects.

Difficulties in describing the mechanism of action of a drug

The mechanism of action of a drug is, at least partially, known from animal pharmacology. However, given the extrapolation issues described above for antidementia agents and the lack of knowledge about the mechanism of the disease to be treated, it is difficult to determine the exact mechanism of action of an antidementia agent. A useful method to help the elucidation of this mechanism in humans is the investigation of the test drug's effects on different levels, from biochemistry and electrophysiology to psychometry, and the analysis of the interrelationship between them. This multi-dimensional assessment will give us a better understanding of the involvement and interaction of the different effect levels and thus increase our understanding of the compound's effects in patients.

Although the difficulties outlined above represent essential problems in the development of antidementia agents, with velnacrine we are in the fortunate position of having results from clinical studies which already demonstrate that this compound has, at least in a major subgroup of patients, significant effects on core symptoms of AD. This is of a two-fold advantage for the task of the present chapter: in retrospect, the efficacy results in patients with AD provide a perspective for the interpretation of the pharmacodynamic effects observed in earlier studies; on the other hand, the pharmacodynamic findings available will help to increase our understanding of the efficacy findings in patients.

PHARMACODYNAMIC EFFECTS OF VELNACRINE

The investigations summarized below came from studies of the effects of velnacrine on the neurophysiological, cerebral blood flow and metabolism and psychomotor/cognitive effect levels. In the first part of this chapter, acute effects after single oral doses of velnacrine are described; the second part will deal with repeated dose effects and their correlation with a response criterion used in the clinical efficacy studies.

Acute effects after single oral doses of velnacrine

Effects of velnacrine on spontaneous EEG and evoked potentials in young healthy subjects

The first pharmacodynamic study conducted with velnacrine in young healthy volunteers investigated the effects of a single oral dose of 100 mg, relative to placebo, on the spontaneous EEG and auditory evoked potentials in 12 young healthy subjects (Kleindienst-Vanderbeke *et al.*, 1987). Despite a large number of variables tested, there was only a clear effect found on the N1 component of the auditory evoked potentials, and this occurred 1.5 hours after medication. No statistically significant effect was observed in the spontaneous EEG.

Ability of velnacrine to antagonize the cognitive deterioration induced by scopolamine in young healthy volunteers

Studies of the effects of scopolamine on cognitive functions played a major role in the history of the central cholinergic deficit hypothesis of AD (see above). This was the reason for testing velnacrine in the 'scopolamine dementia model' in young healthy subjects.

The trial was conducted by Cognitive Drug Research (CDR) Ltd in Reading, UK (see Wesnes *et al.*, 1990). It was designed as a split-plot, double-blind cross-over comparison of two single oral doses of velnacrine (100 mg; 150 mg) and placebo (4×4 Latin square design). One group of subjects ($n1 = 17$) received a dose of 0.4 mg s.c. and the other ($n2 = 14$) 0.6 mg s.c. of scopolamine prior to the administration of either velnacrine or placebo. Outcome variables were a set of cognitive performance tests, assessed by a microcomputerized cognitive test battery (Wesnes, 1985; Wesnes *et al.*, 1987; Simpson *et al.*, 1989), and mood variables measured by the Bond–Lader Visual Analogue Scales (Bond and Lader, 1974). The cognitive test battery mainly consisted of measures of recognition and recall tasks (supra-span lists of words or pictures), measures of the speed of psychomotor coordination (simple and choice reaction time tasks) and various tests of vigilance and attention. Drug effects were evaluated by analyses of variance with two repeated-measurement factors, 'treatment' (100 mg and 150 mg velnacrine, placebo) and 'time' (various measuring points after administration of either velnacrine or placebo).

Generally, the effects of velnacrine were more consistent and pronounced in the subject group with the highest dose of scopolamine (i.e. 0.6 mg s.c.). This was because in this group the impairment of cognitive functions was more severe and showed a less rapid spontaneous recovery under placebo. In two of the three memory tests (immediate verbal recall); delayed word recognition), velnacrine was found to be significantly superior to placebo in reversing the deterioration effects of scopolamine. Similar but less consistent trends were found in the other cognitive tests. In addition, velnacrine improved the mood aspects assessed by the Bond–Lader Visual Analogue Scale, namely feelings of alertness, calmness and contentment.

Acute effects of velnacrine in patients with Alzheimer's disease

A pharmacodynamic study of the acute effect of single oral doses of velnacrine in patients with AD was carried out at the MRC Brain Metabolism Unit of the Royal Edinburgh Hospital (Ebmeier et al., 1992). Patients selected for this study met the DSM-IIIR criteria for dementia (American Psychiatric Association, 1987) and the NINCDS–ADRDA criteria for Probable Alzheimer's Disease (McKhann et al., 1984). The study consisted of two parts. Part one was a double-blind placebo-controlled cross-over study (Latin square design) of single doses of velnacrine (50 mg and 75 mg), physostigmine (2 mg) and placebo. The physostigmine dose chosen was found to be effective in a trial published in the literature (Beller et al., 1975). The outcome measures were two supra-span recognition tasks, a word (12 original words/12 distractor words) and an object (14 original pictures/14 distractors) recognition task. The second part of the study was considered a pilot project. Effects of a single oral dose of 75 mg velnacrine on regional cerebral blood flow were measured by SPECT (single positron emission computed tomography) techniques (comparison: before administration of the drug and 2 hours after administration). Patients were imaged with a Novo 810 scanner or a SME Multimax 810 scanner. Blood flow was examined with ^{99m}Tc-exametazime. The reference region for the evaluation of (relative) changes in regional cerebral blood flow was the calcarine cortex (for details see Bemeier et al., 1992). Thirteen patients were included in this trial. Analysable data were available for 12 patients for the first and 11 patients for the second part of the study. Their Folstein Mini-Mental Total Score had a median of 16; most patients had a 'moderate cognitive decline' according to the Reisberg Global Deterioration Scale (GDS: Reisberg et al., 1982).

The results can be summarized as follows. The object recognition task turned out to be too easy, showing a ceiling effect which made differentiation of drug effects impossible. In the word recognition task, however, there was a significant improvement after 75 mg of velnacrine ($p<0.04$), relative to 50 mg velnacrine and physostigmine which were equivalent to placebo. In the

Rosen, W.G., Mohs, R.C. and Davis, K.L. (1986). Longitudinal changes: cognitive, behavioral and affective patterns in Alzheimer's disease. In: Poon, L.W. (Ed.), *Clinical Memory Assessment of Elderly Adults*. American Psychological Association, Washington, DC.

Sebban, C. (1989). Quantified EEG: a possible tool for classification of SDAT and prediction of drug effects on cognition. *Arch. Gerontol. Geriatr.*, **1** (Suppl.), 237–240.

Siegfried, K.R. (1991). Some considerations on the methodology of clinical trials with potential anti-dementia compounds in patients with Alzheimer's disease. In: Hindmarch, I., Hippius, H. and Wilcock, G. (Eds), *Dementia: Molecules, Methods and Measures*. Wiley, Chichester, New York.

Simpson, P.M., Wesnes, K. and Christmas, C. (1989). A computerised system for the assessment of drug-induced performance changes in young, elderly and demented populations. *Br. J. Clin. Pharmacol.*, **27**, 711–712.

Thal, L.J. and Fuld, P.A. (1983). Memory enhancement with oral physostigmine in Alzheimer's disease. *N. Engl. J. Med.*, **308**, 720.

Thal, L.J., Fuld, P.A., Masur, D.M. and Sharpless, N.S. (1983). Oral physostigmine and lecithin improve memory in Alzheimer's disease. *Ann. Neurol.*, **13**, 491–496.

Wesnes, K. (1985). A fully automated psychometric test battery for human psychopharmacology. *Fourth World Congress of Biological Psychiatry, Philadelphia, September.*

Wesnes, K. and Simpson, P. (1988). Can scopolamine produce a model of the memory deficits seen in aging and dementia? In: Gruneberg, M.M., Morris, P.E. and Sykes, R.N. (Eds), *Practical Aspects of Memory: Current Research and Issues Vol. 2*. Wiley, Chichester, New York.

Wesnes, K., Simpson, P. and Christmas, C. (1987). The assessment of human information processing abilities in psychopharmacology. In: Hindmarch, I. and Stonier, P.D. (Eds), *Human Psychopharmacology. Measures and Models, Vol. 1*. Wiley, Chichester, New York.

Wesnes, K., Simpson, P., Christmas, C. and Siegfried, K. (1990). Effects of HP029 in a scopolamine model of aging and dementia. In: *Abstracts of the 17th CINP (Collegium Internationale Neuropsychopharmacologicum) Congress. Kyoto (Japan). 13–14 September.*

White, P., Hiley, C., Goodhardt, M.J., Keet, J.P., Rrasco, C.A., Bowen, D.M. and Williams, I.A.I. (1977). Neocortical cholinergic neurons in elderly people. *Lancet*, **i**, 669–670.

17

Future Research: Direction and Strategies

GORDON K. WILCOCK

Professor of Care of the Elderly, Frenchay Hospital, University of Bristol, UK

INTRODUCTION

Alzheimer's disease has been the focus of considerable research interest in the last 20 years or so and enormous strides have been made in our understanding of the basic pathology and its therapeutic potential. This is now beginning to be translated into potentially exciting therapeutic strategies and hypotheses. Gone are the days of vasodilators or metabolic enhancers for the treatment of senile dementia or what has also been described as organic brain failure. Currently knowledge allows us to separate out with a considerable degree of certainty, even during life, the differing causes of dementia in both young and older people and target specific strategies to the individual pathologies.

Our initial attempts at treating Alzheimer's disease, although as yet in their infancy, are of course based upon an understanding of the neurotransmitter deficits that are caused in the brain by the disease process, using an approach that is analogous to that of the treatment of Parkinson's disease. Future therapeutic developments however must also address the problem of cell death and malfunction in the hope of slowing down or retarding progression of the illness. One day it may be possible to prevent it altogether but I feel that this is some way off. Until then it is important that we do not forget the need for symptomatic relief in those people who are already showing signs of the illness. This will of course be the majority of sufferers since we rely upon the detection of symptoms to make the diagnosis. This chapter will nevertheless deal only briefly with neurotransmitter-related strategies before moving on to the exciting field of neurotrophic support, and other areas such as protection of the brain from the effects of amyloid, if the latter is indeed toxic, and attempts to try to retard its development.

203

NEUROTRANSMITTER-RELATED STRATEGIES

It has been well known for some time that the ravages of Alzheimer's disease affect particularly the medial temporal structures, especially the hippocampus. These structures play a central role in some aspects of memory function and it is accepted that acetylcholine is the neurotransmitter that is probably most centrally involved in this. In the mid 1970s and early 1980s the cholinergic deficit in the brain in Alzheimer's disease was reported and its relationship to the severity of the clinical manifestations and the pathology firmly established (Perry et al., 1978; Wilcock and Esiri, 1982; Wilcock et al., 1982). The cholinergic hypothesis of Alzheimer's disease was born and this led to early attempts at treatment with cholinergic precursors, e.g. lecithin and choline, the use of a muscarinic agonist such as arecoline in an attempt to enhance the efficacy of acetylcholine at one of its major classes of receptor, and early trials with physostigmine and other anticholinesterases. While some of these approaches, most notably the use of physostigmine and possibly arecoline, led to minor improvements in cognitive performance, there was little if any evidence of significant clinical improvement with any of these agents and certainly nothing of relevance to the day to day life of a sufferer with Alzheimer's disease, or his or her family. The cholinergic hypothesis began to fall into disrepute and a search for other avenues of therapeutic relevance began. In the mid 1980s however the paper by Summers et al. (1986) rekindled interest in the cholinergic hypothesis with their report of a very significant benefit to some patients with Alzheimer's disease when they were treated with a mixture of an anticholinesterase, tetrahydroaminoacridine (THA; tacrine) and lecithin. Many of the early attempts to replicate these findings produced disappointing results but it is now becoming clear, particularly with the publication of some of the more recent trials (Eagger et al., 1991; Davis et al., 1992; Farlow et al., 1992) that the aminoacridines may indeed have something to offer a proportion of sufferers with Alzheimer's disease even if toxicity has to be very carefully monitored. In this respect at least it would appear that we may have our feet on the bottom rung of the ladder of early symptomatic treatment for people suffering from Alzheimer's disease. This is an approach that should not be abandoned but rather refined and coupled with our knowledge of the other neurochemical abnormalities in this condition. For the time being, at least, the development of such strategies is essential for the treatment of established disease symptoms, and we have a long way to go before we will have therapy that is as effective in Alzheimer's disease as are our treatments for people with Parkinson's disease.

A multiplicity of neurotransmitter pathologies exist in Alzheimer's disease, but less attention has been paid to these. Serotonergic and noradrenergic neurochemical pathology is likely to be equally important, particularly as the disease advances, as is the loss of some of the neuropeptides and some of the changes in excitatory amino acid levels. It is also probable that in at least a subgroup of people with Alzheimer's disease the cholinergic deficit is not as important as that of some of the other transmitters (Wilcock *et al.*, 1988).

NEUROTROPHIC FACTORS AND ALZHEIMER'S DISEASE

Nerve growth factor

The neuronal systems that are responsible for the production of many of the neurotransmitters that are depleted in Alzheimer's disease are, at least to some extent, dependent upon one or more trophic factors for the preservation of their functional and structural integrity. This understanding forms the background to the development of therapeutic strategies based on these neurotrophic factors, of which nerve growth factor (NGF) has probably been most explored. This was first identified some 40 years ago by Levi-Montalcini when she and her co-workers reported that mouse sarcomas transplanted into chick embryos induced innervation by sensory and sympathetic fibres. The factor responsible for this was isolated and discovered to be what we now know as NGF. For further information about this early work the reader is referred to a review by Levi-Montalcini (1987).

NGF is a dimeric peptide widely conserved in nature with a very similar structure in each species. In evolutionary terms it has probably played an important part in the development of the central nervous system and a number of studies have now confirmed its neuroprotective role in respect of the survival of cholinergic neurones. The majority of these neurones lie in the basal forebrain, i.e. the basal nucleus of Meynert and the diagonal band of Broca, and are the cells that produce most of the brain's acetylcholine. They show colocalization of antibodies to the NGF receptor and also to cholinergic markers. In addition, physical or chemical ablation of the cortical areas to which the subcortical structures project, or damage to the efferent pathways from these subcortical sites leads to degeneration of the cholinergic neurones at these sites, but this is prevented or reduced by the co-administration of NGF (Gage *et al.*, 1988; Hagg *et al.*, 1988). Similarly, the apparently normal atrophy of cholinergic neurones which is thought to contribute to the impairment of spatial memory in ageing rodents and primates can be improved when NGF is infused into the brain (Fischer *et al.*, 1987; Tuszyinski *et al.*, 1990). Although there does not appear to be a loss of NGF in the cortex of people with Alzheimer's disease (Allen *et al.*, 1991), whether or not NGF is depleted from the subcortical sites is as yet undetermined. There may be a breakdown of intraneuronal transport of NGF from its site of synthesis in the cortex and hippocampus back to the subcortical cholinergic neurones. Whatever is the case, the previously described neuro-protective effect may indicate a therapeutic role in neurodegenerative disorders. Indeed, a recent report (Olson *et al.*, 1992) of the administration of NGF into the ventricular system in the brain of a severely affected Alzheimer's disease sufferer has been interpreted as showing a minor degree of potential benefit and the need for further evaluation of this approach in less affected individuals.

Other neurotrophic factors

It is now clear that there is a whole family of related compounds with neurotrophic effects. These include, in addition to NGF, brain derived neurotrophic factor (BDNF), neurotrophin-3 (NT-3), NT-4 and NT-5. Of these, preliminary evidence indicates that BDNF may be most relevant to Alzheimer's disease. Its mRNA distribution correlates most closely with that seen for NGF and it has been shown to have a neuroprotective effect on rats' septal neurones grown in culture (Philips *et al.*, 1990; Alderson *et al.*, 1990).

Each of these neurotrophic factors binds to both a low affinity and a high affinity receptor. The low affinity receptors appear to be relatively non-specific, e.g. NGF, BDNF and NT-3 appear to bind equally, but the high affinity receptors show greater specificity. The structural homology between these neurotrophic peptides and the physiological properties of their receptors indicate potential therapeutic avenues, and these are currently being explored. At present the therapeutic potential, if this is confirmed, of such an approach would appear to be dependent upon intraventricular administration, with all its attendant problems. Investigation of the structure/function properties of the different peptides may well lead to the development of smaller molecules with the ability to penetrate the blood–brain barrier. If successful, such strategies could slow the progression of Alzheimer's disease by retarding the cell death at sub-cortical sites. Similar strategies may also be relevant to some of the other neurotransmitter systems.

MODIFICATION OF THE AMYLOID RELATED PATHOLOGY

The central role of amyloid in the histological appearance of the brain in Alzheimer's disease is well known. It is present in the plaques that are found in some parts of the brain and also in the walls of some blood vessels, and accumulations of amyloid material are also found scattered diffusely within the brain parenchyma. The amyloid, also known as the ß/A$_4$ peptide, ß-amyloid or amyloid ß-protein is formed from the breakdown product of a much larger protein, amyloid precursor protein (APP) which exists in at least three different isoforms. The APP consists of a long N-terminal segment lying extra-neuronally with a transmembrane segment and a shorter C-terminal portion that lies intracytoplasmically. A small peptide, consisting of approximately 40 amino acid residues, including part of the transmembrane domain, is the sub-unit from which the amyloid itself is assembled.

APP is widely conserved in different species and is indeed also synthesized outside the central nervous sytem. The exact source of the amyloid that is found in the brain in Alzheimer's disease is unclear. It may arise elsewhere in the body, or intrinsically within the brain. If the latter is indeed the case then there are two potential routes of synthesis. One is secretion of the APP from the cell surface, although it would be difficult to explain how the transmembrane portion of the amyloid peptide would be cleaved with the rest of the fragment. It is more likely that the peptide is the product of APP metabolism elsewhere within the neurone, particularly through an endolysosomal pathway.

Amyloid has been assumed to be neurotoxic. Experimental work has shown that at high doses it is indeed toxic to cultured rat neurones (Yankner et al., 1989) but that at low doses it may enhance the survival of such neurones. The neurotoxicity has been shown to be inhibited by tachykinin neuropeptides such as substance P (Kowall et al., 1991). Koh and colleagues (1990) have also reported that the amyloid may increase the toxicity of excitatory amino acid transmitters, especially glutamate. This has been confirmed by others working with cultured human neurones (Mattson et al., 1992). The latter authors however discovered no direct toxicity of amyloid on their cultured human neurones.

It is now clear that the amyloid peptide can occur in the absence of Alzheimer's disease. It has for instance been isolated in a soluble form from cerebrospinal fluid and the blood of healthy people (Seubert et al., 1992). It is probable that the soluble form is a normal metabolite but that the highly insoluble filaments that aggregate in Alzheimer's disease are pathogenic.

Apart from the therapeutic potential of molecules such as substance P and its analogues, where does this knowledge take us in the development of potential therapy? At the moment this is a complex and controversial issue. One approach might be to influence the endolysosomal breakdown pathway and this has been suggested as a potential therapeutic target. Chloroquine is concentrated in lysosomes and has been shown to inhibit the breakdown of APP (Caporaso et al., 1992).

HETEROGENEITY OF ALZHEIMER'S DISEASE

Finally a word about the nosology of Alzheimer's disease. It is clear that what we call Alzheimer's disease is unlikely to be a single condition.

Clinically there are subgroups, histologically there are subgroups and this seems to be mirrored therapeutically since some patients appear to respond to aminoacridines while many do not. It may be too simplistic to expect a single, or related group, of therapeutic strategies to be the answer to all sufferers of Alzheimer's disease. The diagnostic and pathological substrate of this heterogeneity needs to be addressed urgently in the light of the burgeoning number of therapeutic hypotheses.

CONCLUSION

In conclusion, there does appear to be light at the end of the therapeutic tunnel for Alzheimer's disease. What was, only a few years ago, regarded as a task with a relatively hopeless prospect of successful outcome has stimulated much scientific endeavour, which is beginning to bear fruit. We must not forget however that, at least for the present, the diagnosis of Alzheimer's disease depends on the presence of symptoms. Symptomatic treatment based on neurotransmitter related strategies remains important, and research and development in this field is complementary to the other avenues that are being explored.

REFERENCES

Alderson, R.F., Alerman, A.L., Barde, Y.-A. and Lindsay, R.M. (1990). Brain-derived neurotrophic factor increases survival and differentiated functions of rat septal cholinergic neurons in culture. *Neuron*, **5**, 297–306.

Allen, S.J., MacGowan, S.H., Treanor, J.J.S., Feeney, R., Wilcock, G.K. and Dawbarn, D. (1991). Normal NGF content in Alzheimer's disease cerebral cortex and hippocampus. *Neurosci. Lett.*, **131**, 135–139.

Caporaso, G.L., Gandy, S.E., Buxbaum, J.D. and Greengard, P. (1992). Chloroquine inhibits intracellular degradation but not secretion of Alzheimer beta/A4 amyloid precursor protein. *Proc. Natl Acad.Sci. USA*, **89**, 2252–2256.

Davis, K.L., Thal, L.J., Gamzu, E.R., Davis, C.S., Woolson, R.F., Gracon, S.I., Drachman, D.A., Schneider, L.S., Whitehouse, P.J., Hoover, T.M., Morris, J.C., Kawas, C.H., Knopman, D.S., Earl, N.L., Kumar, V., Doody, R.S. and the Tacrine Collaborative Study Group (1992). A double-blind, placebo-controlled multicentre study of tacrine for Alzheimer's disease. *N. Engl. J. Med.*, **327**, 1253–1259.

Eagger, S.A., Morant, N.J. and Levy, R. (1991). Parallel group analysis of the effects of tacrine versus placebo in Alzheimer's disease. *Dementia*, **2**, 207–211.

Farlow, M., Gracon, S.I., Hershey, L.A., Lewis, K.W., Sadowsky, C.H. and Dolan-Ureno, J. for the Tacrine Study Group (1992). A controlled trial of tacrine in Alzheimer's disease. *J. Am. Med. Assoc.*, **268**, 2523–2529.

Fischer, W., Wictorin, A., Bjorklund, A., Williams, L.R., Varon, S.K. and Gage, F.H. (1987). Amelioration of cholinergic neuronal atrophy and spatial memory impairment in aged rats by NGF. *Nature*, **329**, 65–67.

Gage, F.H., Armstrong, D.M., Williams, L.R. and Varon, S. (1988). Morphological response of axotomised septal neurones to nerve growth factor. *J. Comp. Neurol.*, **269**, 147–155.

Hagg, T., Manthorpe, M., Vahlsing, H.L. and Varon, S. (1988). Delayed treatment with nerve growth factor reverses the apparent loss of cholinergic neurons after acute brain damage. *Exp. Neurol.*, **101**, 303–312.

Koh, J.Y., Yang, L.L. and Cotman, C.W. (1990). Beta-amyloid protein increases the vulnerability of cultured cortical neurons to excitotoxic damage. *Brain Res.*, **533**, 315–320.

Kowall, N.W., Beal, M.F., Busciglio, J., Duffy, L.K. and Yankner, B.A. (1991). An *in vivo* model for the neurodegenerative effects of beta amyloid and protection by substance P. *Proc. Natl Acad. Sci. USA*, **88**, 7247–7251.

Levi-Montalcini, R. (1987). The nerve growth factor: thirty-five years later. *Eur. Mol. Biol. Org. J.*, **6**, 1145–1154.

Mattson, M.P., Cheng, B., Davis, D., Bryant, K., Lieberburg, I. and Rydel, R.E. (1992). Beta-amyloid peptides destabilize calcium homeostasis and render human cortical neurons vulnerable to excitotoxicity. *J. Neurosci.*, **12**, 376–389.

Olson, L., Nordberg, A., von Holst, H., Backman, L., Ebendal, T., Alafuzoff, I., Amberla, K., Hartvig, P., Herlitz, A., Lilja, A., Lundqvist, H., Langstrom, B., Meyerson, B., Persson, A., Viitanen, M., Winblad, B. and Seiger, A. (1992). Nerve growth factor affects ^{11}C-nicotine binding, blood flow, EEG and verbal episodic memory in an Alzheimer patient (case report). *J. Neural. Transm. Park. Dis. Dement. Sect.*, **4**, 79–95.

Perry, E.K., Tomlinson, E.G., Blessed, G., Bergmann, K., Gibson, P.H., Perry, R.H. (1978). Correlation of cholinergic abnormalities with senile plaques and mental test scores in senile dementia. *Br. Med. J.*, **ii**, 1457–1459.

Philips, H.S., Hains, J.M., Laramee, G.R., Rosenthal, A. and Winslow, J.W. (1990). Widespread expression of BDNF but not NT-3 by target areas of basal forebrain cholinergic neurons. *Science*, **250**, 290–295.

Seubert, P., Vigo-Pelfrey, C., Esch, F., Lee, M., Dovey, H., Davis, D., Sinha, S., Schlossmacher, M., Whaley, J., Swindlehurst, C., McCormack, R., Wolfert, R., Selkoe, D., Lieberburg, I. and Schenk, D. (1992). Isolation and quantification of soluble Alzheimer's beta-peptide from biological fluids. *Nature*, **359**, 325–327.

Summers, W.K., Majovski, L.V., Marsh, G.M., Tachiki, K. and Kling, A. (1986). Oral tetrahydroaminoacridine in long term treatment of senile dementia, Alzheimer's type. *N. Engl. J. Med.*, **315**, 1241–1245.

Tuszyinski, M.H., U, H.S., Amaral, D.G. and Gage, F.H. (1990). Nerve growth factor infusion in the primate brain reduces lesion-induced cholinergic neuronal degeneration. *J. Neurosci.*, **10**, 3604–3614.

Wilcock, G.K. and Esiri, M.M. (1982). Plaques, tangles and dementia—a quantitative study. *J. Neurol. Sci.*, **56**, 343–356.

Wilcock, G.K., Esiri, M.M., Bowen, D.M. and Smith, C.C.T. (1982). Alzheimer's disease: correlation of cortical choline acetyltransferase activity with the severity of dementia and histological abnormalities. *J. Neurol. Sci.*, **57**, 407–417.

Wilcock, G.K., Esiri, M.M., Bowen, D.M. and Hughes, A.O. (1988). The differential involvement of sub-cortical nuclei in senile dementia of Alzheimer's type. *J. Neurol. Neurosurg. Psychiatry*, **51**, 842–849.

Yankner, B.A., Dawes, L.R., Fisher, S., Villa-Komanoff, L., Oster-Granite, M.L. and Neve, R.L. (1989). Neurotoxicity of a fragment of the amyloid precursor associated with Alzheimer's disease. *Science*, **345**, 417–420.

Index